SAVING HEARTS AND KILLING RATS

Karl Paul Link and the Discovery of Warfarin

Other books by Doug Moe:

The World of Mike Royko

*Lords of the Ring: The Triumph and Tragedy
of College Boxing's Greatest Team*

*Uncommon Sense: The Life of Marshall Erdman
(with Alice D'Alessio)*

Surrounded by Reality: The Best of Doug Moe on Madison

Favre: His Twenty Greatest Games

*Good Men: The Lives and Philanthropy of
Irwin A. and Robert D. Goodman*

*Tommy: My Journey of a Lifetime
(with Tommy G. Thompson)*

*Stroke Runner: My Story of Stroke, Survival,
Recovery, and Advocacy (with Eric Sarno)*

*The Right Thing to Do:
Kit Saunders-Nordeen and the Rise of
Women's Intercollegiate Athletics
at the University of Wisconsin and Beyond*

*Moments of Happiness: A Wisconsin Band Story
(with Mike Leckrone)*

PRAISE FOR "SAVING HEARTS AND KILLING RATS"

Once again, author Doug Moe has demonstrated his ability to turn complicated subjects into compelling, awe-inspiring books that are both educational and a joy to read. His latest effort, "Saving Hearts and Killing Rats," about the esteemed, controversial University of Wisconsin biochemist Karl Paul Link, ranks among his best—a gripping account, filled with surprises, from beginning to end.

— Rob Zaleski, longtime Wisconsin journalist and author of "Ed Garvey Unvarnished" and "David Couper: Beyond the Badge"

With access to family and colleague archives and interviews, and a rare skill for explaining the complex, Moe has fashioned a fascinating—and not always flattering—view of a many-faceted scholar, researcher, mentor, and as it turns out, unshakable humanitarian. This narrative collage manages to combine Stalin, calf nutrition, Eisenhower, patent fights, clover, peace rallies, and an old station wagon into an unvarnished view of Karl Paul Link, the king of rat poison and mischievous windmill-tilter extraordinaire.

— George Hesselberg, veteran Wisconsin journalist and author of "Dead Lines: Slices of Life from the Obit Beat"

Anyone who has spent time digging into the history of Wisconsin science will have heard at least one of the legendary stories about Karl Paul Link. Doug Moe has done us all a service by digging into the lore and separating fact from fiction. Turns out there's more truth than many of us might have thought, and Doug's telling of the tale is just as entertaining as Link himself...well, almost!

— Kevin Walters, historian, Wisconsin Alumni Research Foundation

Karl Paul Link was a brilliant, flamboyant, free-thinking University of Wisconsin biochemist whose discoveries helped save millions of human lives and killed as many rats. It would take a biographer of great depth and breadth to weave together the scientific, personal, and political strands of his life and work. Fortunately, Doug Moe is more than up to the task, producing this lively and engrossing tale of a man who mattered.

— Stuart Levitan, Madison journalist and historian, author of "Madison in the Sixties"

SAVING HEARTS AND KILLING RATS

Karl Paul Link and the Discovery of Warfarin

DOUG MOE

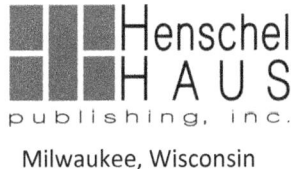

Milwaukee, Wisconsin

Copyright © 2025 by Doug Moe
All rights reserved.

Photographs as credited.

Published by
HenschelHAUS Publishing, Inc.
Milwaukee, Wisconsin
www.henschelHAUS.books.com

ISBN (paperback): 9798991279147
ISBN (hardcover): 9798992107036
LCCN: 2024948261

Printed in the United States of America.

For Tom Link

Table of Contents

1. Farmer Carlson 1
2. La Porte 15
3. Madison 32
4. In Scotland, Success and Controversy 43
5. Elizabeth 63
6. In the Lab 78
7. Dicumarol 93
8. The Road to Warfarin 106
9. Rattor 126
10. Calf Scours and Unpopular Causes 141
11. Warfarin for People 156
12. Less Teaching and Another Lasker 175
13. Doing Good for Mankind 194
14. Endgame 212

Acknowledgements 233
About the Author 237

1. Farmer Carlson

BY ANY MEASURE, THE WINTER of 1932-33 was a terrible season on the Gust Carlson dairy farm, 80 acres in St. Croix County, Wisconsin, some three miles north of Glenwood City.

The Carlson family knew Wisconsin winters by then.

Gust and his young wife, Charlotta, emigrated from Sweden in 1888, departing April 6 for Hull, England, on the SS *Marsdin*. Their infant son Swen was with them.

From Hull, the Carlsons took a train across England to Liverpool, where they caught the SS *Siberian* for Nova Scotia. They docked in Canada April 25 and made their way to Wisconsin.

They lived first on Maple Street in Glenwood City, which at the turn of the century had a population of around 1,700. It was 55 miles east of St. Paul. The Carlsons moved out to the farm in 1904. Theirs was a typically large farm family, seven children in all, including Edwin, born Nov. 30, 1911.

By December 1932, Edwin – Ed to the family – was 21 years old and indispensable on the farm. Gust had turned 70, yet age didn't really matter, everyone worked. On either Monday, Dec. 12 or Tuesday, Dec. 13 – published accounts vary – Charlotta, 64, was doing chores, walking from the milk house to the barn, when she slipped on a patch of ice and fractured her hip. Within several days, she developed pneumonia. It worsened through the day Sunday, Dec. 18, and at 11:30 that night, Charlotta died.

Compounding Ed's grief over the loss of his mother was serious trouble with the farm's dairy herd. They lost two young heifers that December, and others weren't doing well. The local veterinarian mentioned the possibility of something called "sweet clover disease," which only confused Ed Carlson. He – and his father before him – had fed their cows sweet clover for years without issue.

But the farm gods weren't done with Carlson. In January, an older cow, one of Ed's favorites, bled to death after a skin puncture on the cow's thigh. Things got worse. On Friday, Feb. 3, two young cows died. Meanwhile, blood seeped from the nose of Carlson's bull. It was a nightmare. That evening, despite bitter cold temperatures and a chance of snow, Carlson resolved to drive to Madison – some 190 miles away – the following morning. He needed answers about his cattle and thought he might get them at the Wisconsin Agriculture Experiment Station at the University of Wisconsin-Madison.

The Madison campus was home to a young scientist who the previous December – the same month Carlson lost his first two cows to mysterious illness – had himself first heard mention of sweet clover disease.

Karl Paul Link was 31 years old that December – he'd turn 32 in January – and had been on the University of Wisconsin campus, on and off, since 1918, when he enrolled as an undergraduate.

Karl grew up in La Porte, Indiana, son of a Missouri Synod Lutheran minister who died when Karl was 12. The family had limited means, but a creative curiosity and self-sufficiency grew in the children, ten in all (an eleventh died at age six weeks). The house had a piano. It was filled with books. "A deep appreciation of literature, poetry and music became part of us," Margaret, the youngest, recalled later. Karl would remember sadness and some tough days growing up, but by his senior year in high school, he had the lead in both class plays.

If finances held him back at all, it may have come with the decision, once he was in Madison, to set his sights on agricultural chemistry rather than medicine. Why Wisconsin? Perhaps because Link's father was born in the state, and his mother

1. Farmer Carlson

admired Robert M. La Follette, the celebrated Wisconsin progressive.

Karl was an excellent student, but a complicated young man. He later put together an extraordinary scrapbook of prose, verse, photography, and line drawings recalling his time as a student in Madison. He called it "Dances from Seven Years."

Karl was subject to bouts of melancholy throughout his life and they appear in his student scrapbook, where he laments "the mania of patriotism" that had supplanted long held liberal leanings on the UW campus.

This early suspicion of "the mania of patriotism" would evolve, for Karl, into a lifelong distrust of authority and regiment. He flaunted convention. Anne Terrio, who spent more than four decades as secretary of the Biochemistry Department at UW-Madison (it was the Department of Agriculture and Chemistry until 1938), recalled living on State Street when she first moved to the city, around 1930. She ate many meals at a cafeteria in the 500 block run by a woman named Miss Brown. Terrio grew fascinated with a man who frequented the cafeteria. He had long black hair and wore white spats, a big flowing cape, and oversized bow tie. A poet, Terrio thought. Then on her first day working at Biochemistry, the man walked in: Karl Paul Link.

"I couldn't wait," Terrio said, "to get back [to the cafeteria] at noon and tell the girls I now knew who this was."

By then – 1930 – Karl had earned both a master's degree and doctorate from UW-Madison, studying under a plant biologist named William E. Tottingham.

"Tottingham was then a professor of biochemistry," said David L. Nelson, himself a longtime UW-Madison professor of agricultural chemistry and perceptive observer of the department in general and Karl in particular.

"Tottingham was a carbohydrate chemist," Nelson said, "so Link became a carbohydrate chemist."

After earning his Ph.D. in 1925, Karl, according to Nelson, "went to Europe and wandered a little bit."

He studied with eminent scientists in Scotland, Austria, and Switzerland, and brought microanalytical equipment with him when he returned to Madison in 1927, some of the first ever to appear on this side of the Atlantic.

Karl was initially made an assistant professor; by 1931 he'd received a five-year appointment as a research professor with lab facilities part of the deal.

"Link initiated," wrote Robert H. Burris in a biographical memoir, "studies on carbohydrate chemistry, and this is the area in which he first established his solid reputation."

David Nelson noted that Karl's career arc appeared to be set, centered on carbohydrate chemistry and the microanalysis he'd learned from studying with the Nobel Prize winner Fritz Pregl in Austria.

"Link started his career looking at onions," Nelson said, "found a compound in onions that protected them from fungal infections, identified it chemically, and was well on his way to being a world-class carbohydrate chemist."

But then:

"Something happened," Nelson said, "that really changed his life."

What happened was that in February 1933, Ed Carlson, the young St. Croix County farmer with the sick cattle, drove to Madison.

It seems almost certain the date was Feb. 4. Telling the story later, as he did often, Karl recalled it was a Saturday, and the only bad weather Saturday that month in Wisconsin – Karl always mentioned the weather when he told the tale – was the first Saturday.

In Madison, the *Wisconsin State Journal* put the weather on its Saturday, Feb. 4 front page, with a story headlined, "Cold, Probable Snow."

The "blizzard" that Karl eventually recalled never seems to have materialized, but the cold was brutal – 14 below zero in Minneapolis, not far from St. Croix County, on Friday night. It

1. FARMER CARLSON

was 40 below in Winnipeg, Manitoba, this in an era, of course, before wind-chill measurements.

Nevertheless, Carlson piled his truck with a dead cow, a milk can of cow's blood, a substantial amount of spoiled sweet clover hay, and drove the 190 or so miles to Madison.

One of Karl's most complete, and colorful, accounts of what happened that day was related in an address he gave on a February day a quarter century later – a Feb. 25, 1958, speech at the New York Academy of Medicine on Fifth Avenue in Manhattan. Karl's talk was part of a program titled "The Historical and Physiological Aspects of Anticoagulants," and in 1959, it was reprinted in the journal *Circulation* under the title, "The Discovery of Dicumarol and Its Sequels."

Karl noted that he first heard about sweet clover disease in cattle in December 1932 while visiting the University of Minnesota, which was interested in hiring him. Various agricultural issues were discussed and Karl was given a booklet recently written by Lee M. Roderick titled, "Livestock Losses from Sweet Clover."

While Karl rejected the overture from Minnesota, he read the booklet and learned Roderick was one of two veterinary pathologists – the other was Frank Schofield – who had been studying mysterious cattle deaths since the early 1920s. They worked independently, Roderick in North Dakota and Schofield in Canada, but their focus was the same. Why were cows bleeding to death?

"The veterinarians," Karl noted in his New York address, concluded "that the cause of the disease was neither a pathogenic organism nor a nutritional deficiency. The origin of the new malady was traced to stacks of sweet clover hay mysteriously gone bad." Roderick and Schofield soon learned it was only wet – improperly cured – sweet clover hay that caused the disease.

Just two months after Karl's Minnesota visit – around noon on Feb. 4, 1933 – 21-year-old Ed Carlson showed up on the Madison campus with what Karl later called "a disaster load" –

the dead cow, the bucket of blood, and the spoiled sweet clover hay.

Carlson was hoping – on the advice of a St. Croix County veterinarian – to seek help from the Wisconsin Agriculture Experiment Station, established by the state Legislature in 1883 to aid in farm research, part of UW-Madison's charter as a land grant university.

But the station was closed that bitter cold Saturday. One can imagine Carlson, desperate, wondering where he might turn.

"Pure chance," Karl noted later, "brought him to the Biochemistry building." (It was then – in 1933 – called the Agricultural Building.)

It was there he met Karl, who was in the company of a graduate student, Eugen Wilhelm Schoeffel, described by Karl as a "volatile" German who came to the United States in 1926 with a degree in agricultural chemistry.

"Dr. Schoeffel was one of my early assistants here," Karl said, in an interview on a radio program produced by the American Chemical Society. "He was involved in practically everything and was always willing to do anything. He was here the day this farmer came in from Deer Park."

It's interesting that Karl recalled the farmer, Ed Carlson, being from Deer Park, which is a village in St. Croix County some 14 miles northwest of Glenwood City. Since the Carlson farm was itself several miles northwest of Glenwood City, it's likely the farmer described its location to Karl as being between Deer Park and Glenwood City. And indeed Karl, in telling the story in New York City, referred to Carlson as being from "the vicinity" of Deer Park.

On that Saturday in February 1933, there was little for Karl and Schoeffel to do for Carlson other than commiserate. Karl offered what he knew from his recent reading of Roderick's "Livestock Losses from Sweet Clover." He told the young farmer to stop feeding his cattle the spoiled hay, adding that blood transfusions from healthy cattle – not an inexpensive proposition – could also reverse the disease.

1. FARMER CARLSON

Around 4 p.m., Carlson said his goodbyes and headed back to St. Croix County. He left the cow's blood and spoiled sweet clover with Karl.

"I can still see him take off for home," Karl said, in his 1958 New York City address. "Those 190 miles of drifted roads between our laboratory and his barn must have appeared to him like a treacherous and somber ocean."

If Karl was sad and whimsical watching Carlson drive away, Schoeffel, the German assistant, was indignant.

In the New York City speech, Karl employed what he remembered as Schoeffel's "strongly guttural, very earthy" speech, a mix of English and German, to suggest his assistant's aggrieved state, his deep empathy with the farmer Carlson.

At some point, Karl recalled, Schoeffel began dipping his hands into the bucket of cow's blood Carlson left behind, rubbing them together, an action that inspired more oratory.

"Dere's no clot in dat blut! *BLUT, BLUT, VERFLUCHTES BLUT.*" Karl remembered Schoeffel next quoting a line from Goethe's "Faust."

Karl himself, to be certain, was not unmoved by his meeting with Ed Carlson. "I can assure you its impact on me was immense," he said at one point in the New York lecture.

Karl and Schoeffel, once the German had calmed himself, spent some time in the lab rather helplessly considering the hay and blood Carlson had left behind. Outside, it grew dark.

At 7 p.m., Karl announced he was going home. As Karl prepared to leave, Schoeffel grabbed him by the shoulders and looked him straight in the eye.

"Before you go, let me tell you something," Schoeffel said. "Der is destiny dat shapes our ends, it shapes our ends I tell you."

Karl remembered that moment in an interview some years later. Speaking of Schoeffel, Karl said, "He was quite a philosopher. He was almost a mystic. He said, 'There is a destiny that shapes our ends.' In other words, he thought some force above us, that by design had sent this farmer down to us, and we better bear in mind that this wasn't pure accident. This was some 'X' force out there and we better take it very seriously and pay attention to it."

Karl remembered thinking, "Maybe he's right."

David Nelson felt the impact on Karl of Carlson's visit was profound.

"This appeal," Nelson said, "apparently grabbed Link's attention to the point he decided to change, substantially, the direction of his own research. And to take off after this problem."

The promising career in carbohydrate chemistry was set aside, and so began six years of research in the lab – "a long and arduous trail," in Karl's words – to find what it was in the spoiled sweet clover that caused the cows to bleed to death. They began calling this holy grail the "hemorrhagic agent." It proved highly elusive.

"At times," Karl noted, "the hemorrhagic agent appeared to hover before us like thistle down only to elude us like the will-of-the-wisp."

Karl and his team of laboratory assistants – Harold Campbell, Mark Stahmann, Charlie Huebner, and Ralph Overman – set to work on the sweet clover hay puzzle. It was an exhaustive exercise. Across six years, the team made 10,000 blood coagulation tests. They employed more than 1,000 rabbits, 200 rats and 30 guinea pigs – and used 10,000 pounds of spoiled sweet clover.

It was Harold Campbell, having worked through the night, who around dawn on June 28, 1939, isolated on a microscope slide what turned out to be a crystalline coumarin compound – the hemorrhagic agent.

In his 1958 New York City lecture, Karl said he walked into his lab on the morning of June 28, 1939 and found Campbell asleep on a couch. A custodian, Chet Boyles, was drinking from a bottle of something stronger than water.

"I'm celebrating, Doc," Boyles said. "Campy hit the jackpot."

1. FARMER CARLSON

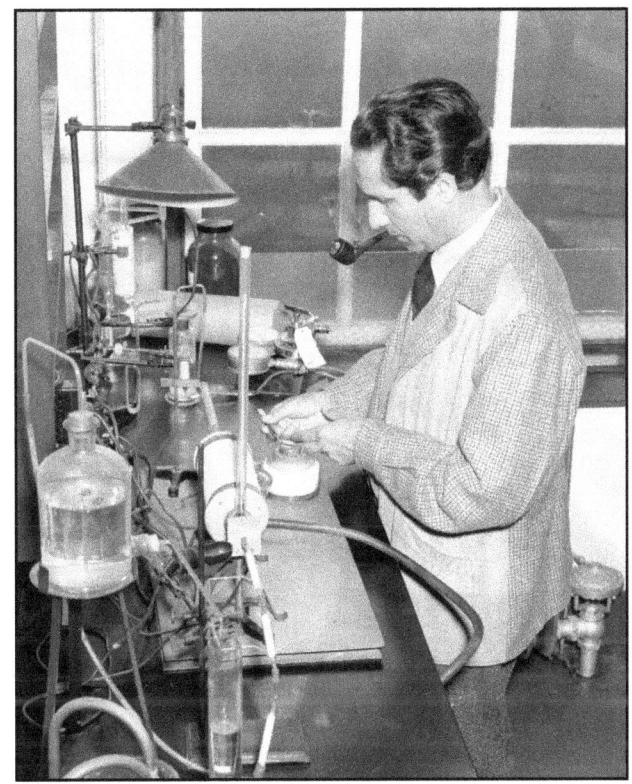

Karl working in his lab. (UW-Madison Archive)

Campbell – unaware that Boyles had leaked his findings – waited two days for the results to be official, then approached Karl in the lab. Campbell held a vial in his hand.

"He was not inclined to show his emotions," Karl recalled, "but it was apparent that he was secretly as happy as a boy who had just caught his first big fish."

Campbell, handing the vial to Karl, said, "This is the H. A.," for hemorrhagic agent.

Karl's team began working with the hemorrhagic agent and then Charlie Huebner and Mark Stahmann synthesized a chemically identical synthetic, achieving it, Karl noted wryly, on April Fool's Day, 1940.

The University of Wisconsin announced the discovery in fall 1940. In hindsight, the general response seems muted. A short article ran on page three in the Madison *Capital Times* on a

Saturday afternoon in November 1940, under the headline: "Solve Mystery of Disease in Cattle."

Of course, they had done much more than that. It was teased in the last paragraph of the story:

"Although the toxic coumarin compound [in spoiled sweet clover] causes mischief on the farm, there is at least a possibility that it may prove useful in medicine if it affects man as it does most animals. Because it is very potent in preventing the coagulation of blood, it may have value in diseases caused or complicated by blood clots."

It didn't stay muted long.

Over the next two decades, Karl Paul Link became famous. Early on, the synthetic compound – called dicumarol – was tested for use as an anticoagulant in humans, with attendant press reports. A more potent version, named warfarin – a combining of the Wisconsin Alumni Research Foundation (WARF) – which assisted the scientists with patenting and licensing – and coumarin, was used first as a highly effective rodenticide, and then an anti-clotting agent that doctors famously prescribed for President Dwight Eisenhower after his 1955 heart attack. Today an estimated 100 million prescriptions for warfarin are issued each year.

Karl was invited to speak at the Mayo Clinic in 1942 – the first time he told the farmer Ed Carlson story to a wide audience – and was elected to the National Academy of Sciences in 1946. In 1952, when he was awarded the Cameron Prize by the University of Edinburgh in Scotland, an article in *The Capital Times* referred to Karl as "internationally famed." By 1960, he had twice received the prestigious Lasker Award – often a precursor to the Nobel – "for fundamental contributions to our understanding of the mechanics of blood clotting."

If Karl was famous by then, he was also feuding, with among others, Harry Steenbock, a UW colleague whose use of Vitamin D to cure rickets launched WARF while Karl was still in graduate school. Steenbock was an establishment figure who still held great sway with WARF in the 1940s and '50s, neither of which would have endeared him to Link. The two had a physical

1. FARMER CARLSON

altercation in a restroom that spilled out into the hall, assuring it would become mythic in the annals of WARF, which it has. Less well known is a story Anne Terrio, the department secretary, told in a UW Oral History Program interview of a chat she was having with Karl in her office when Steenbock walked in. Such was their dislike that Steenbock, without a word, turned around to leave.

Link picked a ball of twine off a table near where he was sitting and threw it at Steenbock.

Terrio was quick to balance this "childish" action of Link's with her feeling that he was a "essentially a very kind, thoughtful person. He did many, many nice things for people. But every once in a while…"

Another lamentable feud was with Mark Stahmann, Karl's lab assistant in the 1930s, which among other things concerned credit for the lab's anticoagulants. (Both Stahmann's and Karl's names, along with Miyoshi Ikawa, are on the warfarin patent.) Whatever the instigator, the two men – as with Karl and Steenbock – reached a point where they could hardly be in the same room.

Lest anyone conclude that Karl was a less than generous colleague, consider Harold Campbell, who remembered Karl insisting that he – Campbell – find his own way in the lab.

"It was always," Campbell recalled, "'Campy, you can do it. Campy, you can do it. Go.' Encouragement? Yes. Confidence? Yes. But not, 'Campy, why don't you try this next?' As soon as he did this, Karl would have had the experience of… manipulating the experimental method… He might have been successful and… built on his strength in this field."

But it wouldn't have been as beneficial for Campbell.

"I might have been better at following instructions," Campbell noted. "But I wouldn't have had the experience of manipulating the experimental method and making new, creative discoveries."

Karl's repeated jousting with the "establishment" – University of Wisconsin administrators were a favorite target – was often cast in a jocular light. He liked to say that at the same 1952 UW Board of Regents meeting when he was censured over a dispute about his research on calf scours, he was also given a raise. The stories added to Karl's colorful reputation and were often recalled with humor. But there was a seriousness to the disputes, as well, particularly those when Karl, as he often did, spoke up in support of unpopular causes.

Did Karl's personality overshadow his science? Not to Irving S. Wright, an esteemed New York cardiologist who worked with Karl.

"As a scientist," Wright said, "he is deceptive, in the sense that his scientific works are so correct and so conservative, as compared to his general character, as you would judge it to meet him. It's almost a paradox in one man. But he's an extraordinarily brilliant person. For five years, we were co-members of a committee for the setting up of conferences on blood clotting. Dr. Link always kept the meetings in a constant state of ferment, one might almost say uproar, by his unusual approaches and the manner in which he thought in reference to our problems. This was very salutary in my opinion."

The awards, money, fame – Karl wore them all with a winning irreverence. In 1974 – four years before Karl's death – he told his favorite newspaper reporter, the talented John Newhouse of the *Wisconsin State Journal*, a story about having recently attended a dinner at Cambridge University, honoring Dr. A. C. Chibnall, an eminent protein chemist. At one point in the evening, Link asked Chibnall's wife, a Latin scholar, for the Latin translation of something Link was considering for his epitaph: "He gave rats an easy out."

The story Karl told about Ed Carlson coming to Madison with his "disaster load" in 1933 – triggering Karl's groundbreaking work with blood anticoagulants – has been questioned by some. In a biographical memoir of Karl written for the *National Academies Press*, Robert H. Burris noted, "The distance the farmer traveled has increased with the years and the weather at the time of the visit has deteriorated considerably."

1. FARMER CARLSON

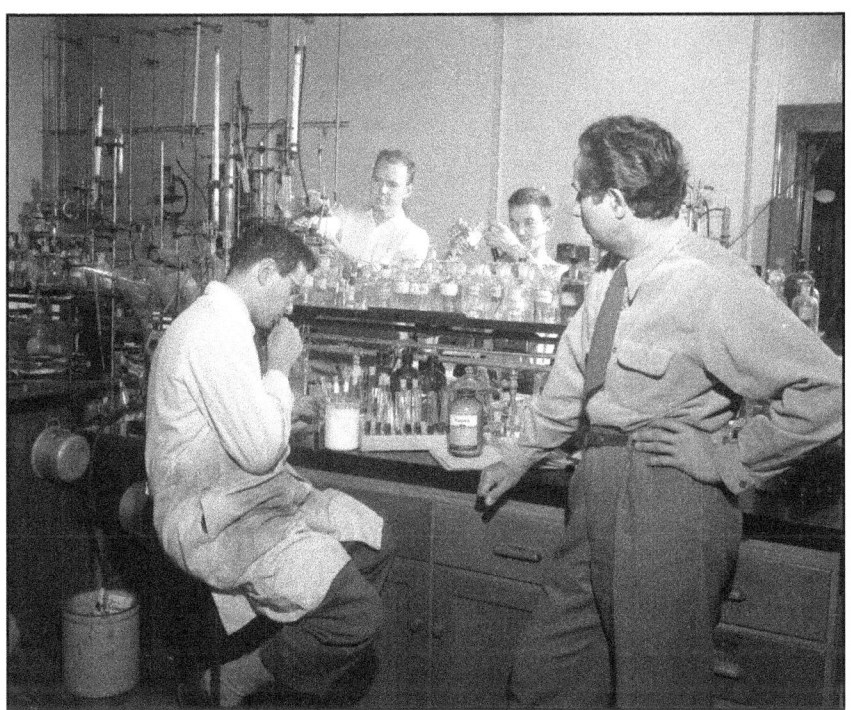

Karl, in foreground, advising his students. Many of his students went on to distinguished scientific careers of their own. (UW-Madison Archive)

Burris wrote that Karl's assistant Mark Stahmann never bought the story, saying, "I distrust direct quotations that are recorded twenty-six years after the fact."

But Link first told the Carlson story to an audience not in 1958 but in 1942, at the Mayo Clinic. And original research for this book was able to confirm that there was a young farmer named Ed Carlson in St. Croix County in 1933. In an American Chemical Society radio interview, Karl mentioned that Carlson's father was also a farmer, which was true – Gust Carlson started the farm in 1904.

A final note of interest in the Carlson story is that Ed Carlson himself may never have realized the important role he played in one of the biggest medical breakthroughs of the 20th century. Ed Carlson died in 1975, at home in St. Croix County. His son, Stanley Carlson, an emeritus professor at the University of Wisconsin-Stevens Point, was recently asked if he knew the story. He did not, reacting to it with amazement. Speaking of his dad, Stanley said, "He never mentioned it."

If the Carlsons were farmers, the Links, going back at least two generations, were ministers. Neither Karl nor any of his nine siblings followed that path, but they all lived fruitful lives.

In a eulogy for Karl in 1978, Saul Roseman observed, "All ten children fashioned successful careers, many of them professionally."

Their parents, Roseman added, "must have been remarkable."

Truth is, it ran throughout the family.

2. LA PORTE

KARL'S GRANDFATHER, GEORG LINK, emigrated from Germany to the United States. He was born in Bavaria in 1829.

"We go back to the 1700s in Germany," said Sandra Lignell, daughter of Karl's older brother, Herbert Link. Sandra studied the Link family history.

Georg Link was part of a wave of young men distrustful of the religious rationalism that was sweeping Germany. Many made their way to the United States.

Georg graduated from the Lutheran Seminary in Fort Wayne, Indiana in 1851. He was a member of the Lutheran Church-Missouri Synod – originally called the German Lutheran Evangelical Church – which had formed four years earlier when 12 pastors representing 16 German Lutheran congregations met in Chicago and expressed their mutual dissatisfaction with much of American Lutheran doctrine. The Missouri Synod was conservative and adhered to the Confessional Lutheranism as contained in the 1580 Book of Concord.

Georg Link became one of its stars.

"One of the most powerful pulpit orators of the German Evan. Lutheran Church," according to a 1908 story in the Edwardsville, Illinois *Intelligencer*. "Possessing exceptional powers of lucid and concise exposition of the scriptures. As a Homilete he had but few equals. He was an author and compiler and was well known among the German Lutherans of the country."

Married in 1854 to Hannah Lange – herself a German immigrant – Georg across half a century held pastorates at more than half a dozen churches in the Midwest, including Lebanon, Wisconsin, the town where Karl's father, George, was born in April 1863.

One of Georg's most notable postings was the 13 years (1873-1886) he spent at Zion Lutheran Church in St Louis, during which time he served four years as vice-president of the Western District of the Lutheran Church-Missouri Synod. It was in Georg's last year in that role – 1877 – that he compiled a book of Martin Luther's best daily devotionals. It was published in German. More than a century later, it was translated by Joel Baseley and published in English, with Georg Link still acknowledged as editor.

Georg spent four years (1888-1892) at the Trinity Evangelical Lutheran Church in Springfield, where he presided over the building of a new church. Georg's son-in-law, Charles Frederick May, was selected as the project architect, though his initial budget of $20,000 was deemed too expensive and redone at a figure of $16,000. The new building was dedicated in late September 1888, with a final crowning touch revealed in the church's September 1, 1888 minutes: "It was resolved that Pastor Link and A. Schuppe be permitted to order two bells for our new church, and to gather subscriptions." The bells were in place for the dedication.

In 1901, Georg celebrated the 50th year of his ordination. There was a party and a small newspaper story headlined, "Fifty Years in the Ministry."

By then, Georg had joined his son, George Link – Karl's father – at the St. John's German Lutheran Church in La Porte, Indiana. Georg was assistant pastor to his son, who arrived in La Porte in 1890. Georg stayed only a year in La Porte, but it was the year, 1901, that he commemorated 50 years in the church, and the year, too, that his grandson Karl was born. Georg soon moved to an assistant pastor's position in Chester, Illinois and then, in 1907, to emeritus pastor status in Springfield. That's where Georg died, September 21, 1908, at age 79. A newspaper story headlined

2. La Porte

"Aged Pastor Is Called" noted that "his declining days were serene and beautiful," and mentioned his fame throughout the Midwest as an orator. It noted that he was survived by his wife, Hannah (who would live another decade), 39 grandchildren, a daughter and two sons, including George.

It appears George was always going to follow his father's path. Born in Lebanon, Dodge County, Wisconsin, a 1913 La Porte newspaper story about George noted: "When still a young lad he had made up his mind to become a minister of the Lutheran church."

George was born in 1863, attended Lutheran school in Lebanon and moved with his family to St. Louis when he was a young teen. He spent three years at the Concordia Academy "taking Latin, scientific and commercial courses," according to the 1913 article. In 1878, he entered Concordia College in Fort Wayne, Indiana. The campus was moved from St. Louis to Fort Wayne in 1861, where it combined with the Practical Theological Seminary.

"He took the regular course at that college," the article notes, "including Latin, Greek, Hebrew and a little French."

In 1882, George returned to St. Louis, enrolling in the Concordia Seminary, the theological university of the Missouri Synod. His theology studies were abetted with philosophy, logic and metaphysics. While a student, George often preached at Lutheran churches in the St. Louis area. Summers he spent as a vicar in Lutheran churches in outposts including Troy, Illinois and North St. Louis.

George graduated from Concordia in 1885. He stayed for several months as a post-graduate, attending lectures, and then in May 1886 accepted a pastor position at a small Lutheran church in Mt. Clemens, Michigan.

Mt. Clemens at the time was best-known for its mineral baths – drawn from nearby springs – which at one time numbered nearly a dozen and drew the wealthy and celebrated. Tourism related to the baths was Mt. Clemens' biggest industry. Babe

Ruth came to town for the baths, and William Randolph Hearst. Belief in the "miracle" powers of the water began to fade by the mid-20th century.

When George Link arrived, in 1886, the first bathhouse in Mt. Clemens was only a little more than a decade old. George may have enjoyed the bath, but pretty quickly his free time was taken up by a young woman, a native of nearby Monroe, Michigan – perhaps best known as the childhood home of General George Armstrong Custer – named Fredericka Mohr.

Like the Links, the Mohrs came to the United States from Bavaria. Fredericka's father, Konrad Mohr, emigrated in 1847.

"He was a stonecutter," Sandra Lignell said. "He had a marble company in Monroe. Most of the old tombstones in the Lutheran cemetery in Monroe were cut and fixed by him."

George and Fredericka married in May 1887, in Monroe, a year after George's arrival in Mt. Clemens.

"She married a Lutheran pastor at 18," wrote their son, Karl Paul Link, in notes for an unpublished memoir. "She was beautiful then."

She was beautiful, but she wasn't 18. Fredericka was 20 on the day of the wedding. She was destined to have 11 children, losing one in infancy. The others lived long lives.

"She was wise, laconic, tough in mind and body," Karl wrote of his mother. "She was very devout."

In another passage devoted to his mother in the memoir notes, Karl wrote: "She lacked the benefit of formal schooling – had to stop at the 4th grade – but was one of the most highly educated women I have known. She always did it, so to speak, by example. She quoted Goethe frequently… and she used to say if it is your good fortune to be well endowed by the Lord, you sin if you do not use that talent for the benefit of mankind in some way or another."

During the early years of the marriage, George served as church pastor in Mt. Clemens and taught five days a week in the church's parochial school.

2. La Porte

In September 1890, the young couple moved to La Porte, Indiana, where George became pastor at St. John's Lutheran Church, established in 1857.

In those four years in Michigan, George had made an impression. The Mt. Clemens newspaper, the *Monitor*, took note: "We congratulate Mr. Link upon his promotion to a much larger field of action, and wish him success, but at the same time we condole with his congregation upon the loss of an able, hardworking and efficient pastor, and with the whole community, upon our loss of a good and useful citizen."

La Porte – hometown of Karl and his siblings – has a rich history. It was visited in the 17th century by French explorers who named the area – site of a wide Pottawatomie Nation trail that stretched between forest and prairie – "La Porte," French for "the door."

La Porte was established as a settlement in 1832 and incorporated as a town three years later. By 1852, the town had 5,000 residents, and La Porte University, whose attendees included William Worrall Mayo, who with his sons later established the famed Mayo Clinic in Minnesota. Less happily, La Porte was also home to Belle Gunness, one of the 19th century's most notorious serial killers, having murdered numerous wealthy men – more than a dozen – for their money in her farmhouse in La Porte.

The 1913 La Porte article on George Link mentioned the thriving congregation he served for a decade at St. John's in La Porte and made statistical reference to that service, noting George performed 778 baptisms, 631 confirmations and 237 marriages.

That record – and remembering how George had wanted to be a Lutheran minister "when still a young lad" – makes what happened in 1899 both shocking and sad. George began to struggle while delivering sermons. Words would fail him, sentences were left unfinished. The 1913 La Porte article described it as "a serious throat condition." George's grandson, Karl's son Tom Link, believes it was likely spasmodic dysphonia, a neurological disorder affecting the voice muscles in the larynx. For someone whose voice equated to his livelihood, it must have been terrifying.

Perhaps the condition came and went, because for a few years, George continued in his ministry. In 1901, his father, Georg, came to La Porte to assist his son. Meanwhile, George and Fredericka's family continued to grow. Their first child, George, was born in 1887. Karl, born in La Porte in 1901, was their eighth. In between were Alfred, Herbert, Helene, Ruth, Theodore, and Agnes. Walter and Margaret would follow Karl.

Physically, Karl was not a robust child.

"That I should have been born so sickly looking wasn't my fault," Karl noted in his memoir notes.

"Mother Link," he continued, "would appear in retrospect was already somewhat worn out. The milk secreting and milk feeding mechanism didn't function. The previous seven had all been fed at her breast." Elsewhere in his notes, Karl mentions that instead of breast milk, he received Horlick's Malted Milk, cod liver oil and malt extract.

"For number eight there was no milk – just concern," Karl wrote. "She was of course always aware of my relatively weak physical make-up... I do recall that I was baptized as promptly as possible in the parsonage."

Before he was two, Karl contracted pneumonia.

"[He was] restored to health with mustard packs and the night-long vigilance of his mother," wrote the journalist Don Behm in a 1979 biographical memoir of Karl. Fredericka would later say that having watched her toddler son survive such a serious illness, she felt he might be destined for something great.

Karl, for his part, later wondered if he hadn't, in infancy, contracted an infection that would bedevil him at various points throughout his life: tuberculosis.

In notes for his memoir, Karl recounts a conversation with a Dr. Dickie:

"I got my first dose in 1901," Karl said, referencing the year of his birth.

2. La Porte

"So you subscribe to the theory that you got the infection as a child?" Dr. Dickie replied.

"I do," Karl said. "And what's more – I got a good-sized dose."

Joan Link Coles, daughter of Karl's younger brother, Walter, said in an interview for this book that there were other instances of tuberculosis in the family, particularly among the sisters. All four eventually moved to the Tucson area, Coles said, "so they could breathe healthy air."

The year of Karl's pneumonia – 1903 – was the year his father, George, stepped away from the church. The throat ailment brought about "serious nervous trouble," according to the 1913 La Porte newspaper article. "He was in fear of losing his mind."

The article continued, "His congregation, which had shown him much love and sympathy, reluctantly accepted his resignation."

George worked for a time as a shipping clerk, and then in March 1904, accepted a position as assistant state agent for the prison in nearby Michigan City, Indiana. He "quickly established the reputation of being the prison's missionary and the paroled man's friend," according to the 1913 La Porte article.

In fall 1904, George was elected clerk of LaPorte County (inexplicably, the county, unlike the city, does not utilize a space in the name LaPorte).

"It was predicted at that time," the 1913 article noted, "that he would make the best clerk the LaPorte circuit had ever had, and this prediction was quickly verified… Mr. Link discharged the duties of his office with painstaking care, and he inaugurated several reforms in office work and office records, all of which saved money for the taxpayer."

Karl attended St. John's Lutheran school in La Porte for eight years prior to entering La Porte High School.

"They went to German Lutheran school," Sandra Lignell, daughter of Karl's brother, Herbert, said. "My father didn't learn to speak English until he went to high school because the first eight grades, everything was in German."

"We spoke both German and English," said Karl's sister, Margaret.

The home at 616 C Street included lively discussions about books, often punctuated by music – someone seated at the piano that came from Germany with Karl's maternal grandparents, the Mohrs.

Karl shared a bedroom on the third floor with three brothers: Theodore, Herbert and Walter. "There were four cubicles with windows," Karl wrote in his memoir notes.

After recalling the living quarters, Karl continued, "It has been said more than once by those who were familiar with the boys of Pastor George Link [that] they are a pugnacious lot. They have to do their arguing on the third floor. When the three elder of the last four Link boys get into a verbal discussion on anything – you're liable to have five or more opinions on almost anything.

"Violence was not tolerated by our parents," Karl continued. "If you didn't like the verbal hassle, you could take a walk."

All the kids had nicknames. They resurfaced in a 1950 Tucson *Daily Citizen* article that was occasioned by a partial reunion of the siblings – including Karl – in Tucson. All four Link sisters, as mentioned, lived in Tucson and Arizona was a nice place to visit in January 1950.

"They still use the pet names developed in childhood," the Tucson story noted, and in addition to mentioning the nicknames, the story also made clear how accomplished the Link siblings were by 1950.

George, the first born, was a distinguished plant pathologist at the University of Chicago. His nickname was "Kuni." Alfred ("Fipps") was a judge. Walter ("Krish") was a geologist with Standard Oil. Herbert ("Tiny") was a government weather observer. Theodore ("Uncle Bim") was a petroleum geologist. Margaret ("Spatz") was executive secretary of the local Red Cross. Agnes ("Rags") was a nurse. Ruth ("Gnatz") was a hat designer and retailer. Helene ("Lane") was a professional musician.

2. La Porte

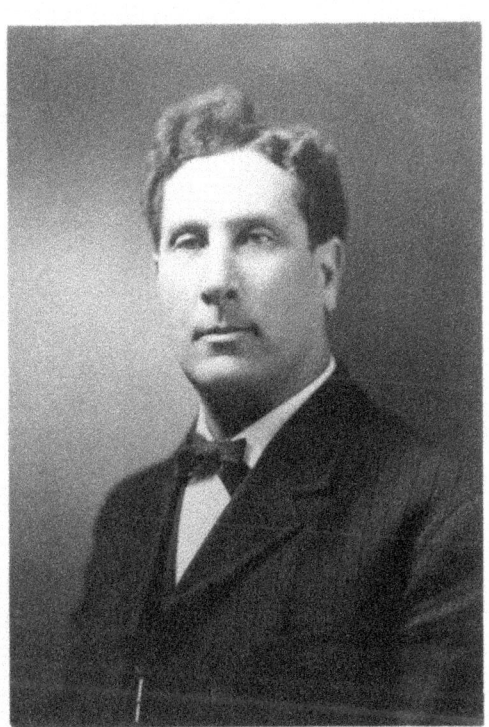

Karl's father, Rev. George Link. (Link family)

Karl, of course, was by 1950 a world-famous biochemist, still known to his siblings as "Chas."

Forty years earlier – in 1910 – the family on C Street in La Porte was on the precipice of a devastating loss. It started when the patriarch, county clerk George Link, fainted in his office. Tests revealed cancer in his colon. He was operated on in February 1911, and again that June. His doctors told the family it was doubtful George would live out the year.

He did, however, and had three more surgeries in 1912.

The 1913 La Porte article that has been quoted several times here – and was titled "Death Claims a Good Man" – offered a glimpse into George Link's final days:

"It was only his great strength and the exceptionally fine care which he had at the hands of his wife, who through all his illnesses ministered to his wants, that kept him alive for nearly a year after the last operation. The suffering which Mr. Link underwent was most excruciating and during much of the time it was necessary to keep him under the influence of opiates. For 17 weeks, he had been in bed all of the time. He was conscious until half an hour before the end came and previous to becoming unconscious he bade his family an affectionate goodbye."

Sometime after midnight on Sept. 12, 1913, George Link convulsed and slipped into unconsciousness. According to the La Porte article, George died at approximately 1:30 a.m.

In his memoir notes, Karl recalled that "official word was passed 2-2:30 a.m." Karl was in bed on the third floor of the C Street house. He didn't cry, explaining that he had cried himself out over the past few days. Twelve-year-old Karl went down to the pantry and looked out the same window from where in May 1910 he had seen Halley's Comet. He wrote later that he looked out the window thinking about his dad and asking questions that had no answer, among them, "Why?"

Before sunrise – it was a mild late summer early morning – Karl went back upstairs and this time looked out a window to the north. In the moonlight, he saw a spotted gray horse pulling a carriage. It stopped at the Link home, and a man, a mortician named Decker, got out and tied the horse to a post.

Soon the family gathered for breakfast while Karl stayed at the third-floor window. His older sister, Agnes, came to retrieve him. She was crying. Karl was not. He refused to leave the window. In her grief, Agnes lashed out.

"You will go to hell if you don't cry – and pray."

"Go away," Karl said. "Leave me alone."

His mother suggested Karl eat something and go back to bed.

Funeral services were held at St. John's Lutheran church and George was buried at Pine Lake Cemetery in La Porte. Years later, Karl remembered little of the service, apart from an uncle singing *"O Haupt Voll Blut und Wunden,"* a Christian passion hymn translated from Latin to German by the Lutheran hymnist Paul Gerhardt.

2. La Porte

George's six sons were pallbearers, in three rows of two. Karl and his brother Walter formed the middle row, with Karl on the right. The hearse was black. It seemed to Karl it took a long time to get to the cemetery, where he recalled the pastor's recitation: "*Erde zu Erde, Asche zu Asche, Staub zu Staub*": "Earth to earth, ashes to ashes, dust to dust."

Karl went to bed early, right after supper, that night. Waking in the morning, he felt a bit better, his 12-year-old mind still filled with questions related to suffering and eternity. Recalling that morning and those questions nearly a half century later – writing in his memoir notes before dawn on March 27, 1959 – Karl concluded, "I do not know!!"

The family found a way of going on.

"The frugality and austerity of the parsonage and house in which I grew up would stagger most of you," Karl wrote later. "There was nothing there to waste: time, food, materials, let alone money. There wasn't any money. Our father had died at 50 – he left his widow with ten children, seven were minors. No insurance. No estate."

Karl's sister, Margaret, was less bleak in her description to Robert H. Burris for his biographical memoir of Karl.

"There was always enough food for the family," Margaret said. "We were adequately clothed wearing 'hand me downs,' given the best toys and of course many books. We often asked each other, how did our mother raise us when there was so little money? When people asked this question of our mother, she would reply with a smile on her face, 'My husband left me with a great heritage, a library with many books, a thirteen-room house without a mortgage, a good reputation, and ten children.'"

Joan Coles, daughter of Walter Link, said her father's description of life on C Street more closely matched Karl's.

"The fact of the matter is they didn't have much at all," Coles said. "They had a very large garden and I think they kept a beehive. They had very limited earnings. All the boys worked."

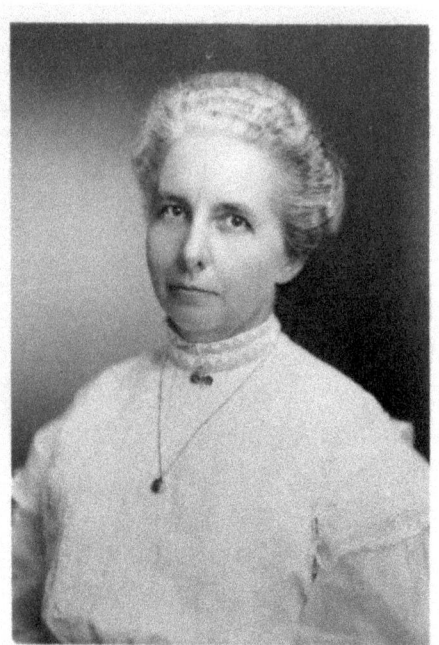

Karl's mother, Fredericka Link. (Link family)

Walter also gave his daughter the impression that their mother – left in a precarious position with the death of her husband, and seven kids in the house – could be distant and demanding. "She ruled with an iron hand," Coles said. "I'm very sure of that."

The teenage Karl was occasionally melancholic – he noted that his mother, aware he was having a bad day, would allow him to stay home from school – but he also recalled, in his memoir notes, good times at the LaPorte County fair and church picnics on the Fourth of July and Labor Day.

Karl also remembered a friend named Billy Walton whose father owned a tobacco store in La Porte. When Billy's father died in 1914, a year after Karl's own father's death, Karl helped Billy move the metal Indian that stood out front of the store to the Walton residence at the south end of La Porte.

Karl admitted to a crush on Mrs. Walton. "She was really beautiful," he wrote, and "did not wear a girdle or brassiere."

2. La Porte

In his memoir notes, Karl concluded, "I was of course too young to make any advances."

Karl's interests at La Porte High School were wide-ranging. The Class of 1918 senior yearbook, titled *The Reflector*, notes that in his junior year he participated in the English club, German club and on the track team. As a senior, Karl played basketball, acted in the class plays and was president of the Boys' Community Garden.

With their yearbook picture, each senior was assigned an unattributed quote that presumably reflected how they were regarded by their peers. Karl's read: "Though vanquished he can argue still." Years later, more than one university administrator would agree.

The Boys' Community Garden first drew the interest of Karl's brother, Walter. He was one of 28 members and served as treasurer when the club was formed in spring 1917, a time when

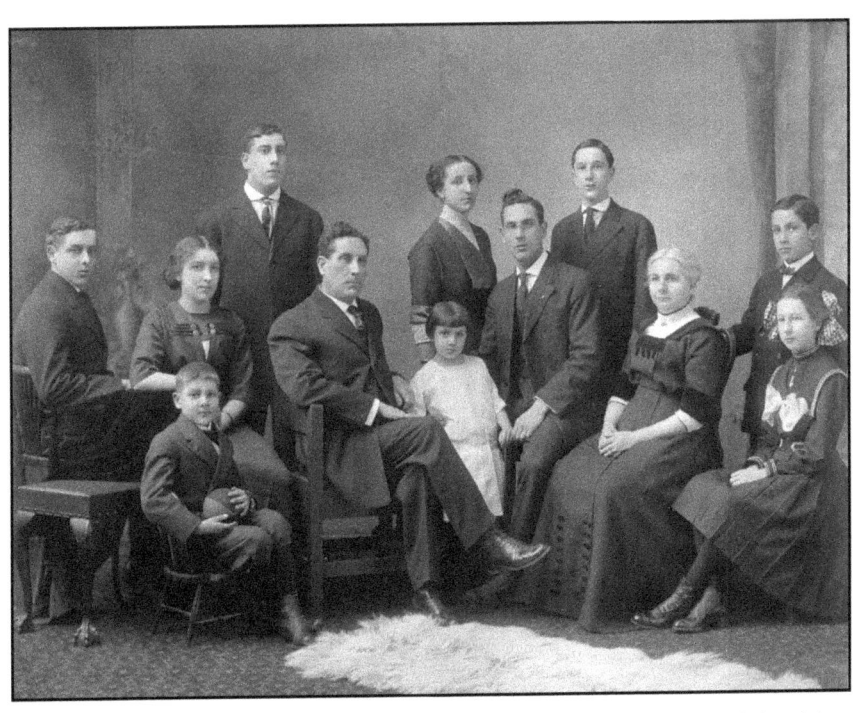

Karl, standing far right, with his parents and siblings, in La Porte. (Link family)

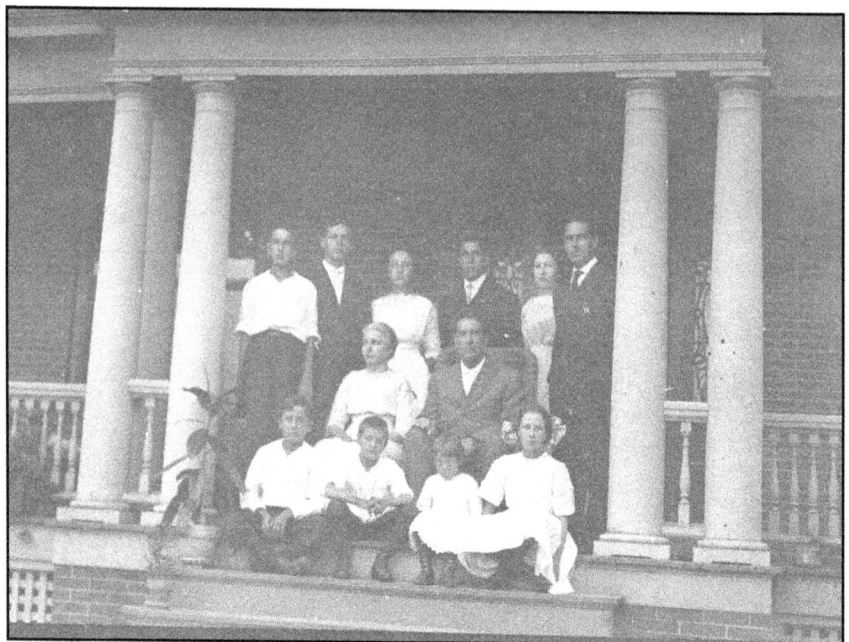

Karl with his parents and his nine siblings,
at their home in La Porte. (Link family)

there was a nationwide call for more farm crops, as the United States was at war. The La Porte Chamber of Commerce rented seven acres of land and donated it for use as the high schoolers' community garden. A botany teacher, Isaac Conner, supervised the growing of potatoes, corn, tomatoes and more.

A year later, the garden was less formalized – the Chamber of Commerce ceased its participation. But Karl stepped up. Seven of the boys – with Karl as president – did a second garden on their own, renting five acres of land. Over the winter, Karl wrote a letter to the University of Wisconsin College of Agriculture asking for advice on certified seed growers.

A letter dated Feb. 18, 1918, came back to Karl's house on C Street from an associate professor of horticulture:

"Dear Sir: Your letter of recent date has just been received. I am enclosing herewith a list of certified seed growers. I would also refer you to Mr. Karl Hazelberg, Secretary, Barron, Wiscon-

2. LA PORTE

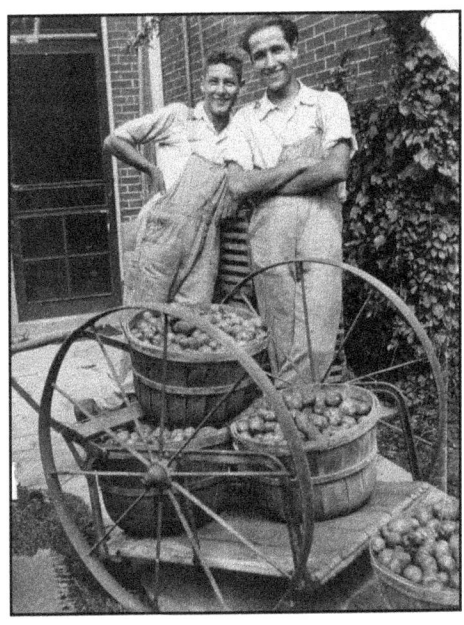

Karl, right, with his younger brother, Walter, in La Porte, with their potato harvest. Crop proceeds helped fund their college education. (Link family)

sin, who is secretary of the Wisconsin Certified Seed Potato Growers Association."

Karl contacted Hazelberg, who on March 20 sent this letter to C Street: "Dear Sir: Your valued order for seed potatoes, with draft enclosed, is at hand. Our price has dropped with the other market therefore we will ship you 150 pounds instead of 120 pounds as ordered."

Karl's predilection for agriculture and livestock was such that it was spoofed in the high school yearbook, in a few pages near the back where a mock La Porte newspaper – dated August 17, 1935 – was displayed.

One of the "news" stories began: "The many friends of Karl Link, the noted stock raiser, will be pleased to learn that he accepted a position with the National Pig raising school of Kansas City, as president and head professor. Mr. Link is a product of the La Porte school having studied under the eminent agriculturalist, Mr. I. L. Conner. It may be said that ever since Mr. Link made his world renown speech on agriculture, before the La Porte High School assembly he has been recognized as an authority on this subject."

More seriously, Karl was clearly an exceptional student. He was one of two seniors chosen to represent La Porte in May 2018 at the University of Chicago's Chicago Competitive Examination, an opportunity for high school seniors to win college scholarship prizes. Karl was examined in German and History. The yearbook did not reveal whether he received scholarship funds but noted Karl and his classmate "reported a fine time, appreciating the value of the examinations, and the hospitality of the University."

Karl had one more passion in high school: acting.

"I confess the art of showmanship comes easy to all the Link boys," Karl wrote, many years later, "since their father [was] from 1890 till 1905 [actually 1903] probably as good an orator in the Missouri Lutheran Synod in Northern Indiana as any."

In January 1918, Karl had first billing in the senior class production of "It Pays to Advertise," a three-act farce in which Karl played a soap magnate whose son attempts to undermine him by opening a rival enterprise. It played to 650 people at the Central School Auditorium and was well enough received that the students were asked to present it again a month later as a benefit for the Red Cross.

That spring, the senior class mounted "The County Chairman," a 1903 comedy written by George Ade. Karl played the county chairman of the title.

For college, Karl chose the University of Wisconsin in Madison. His older brothers who attended college – George, Alfred and Theodore – all enrolled in the University of Chicago. No direct statement from Karl about this choice appears to exist, though a 1948 Madison *Capital Times* story, for which Karl was interviewed, noted the following:

"Because of Wisconsin's liberal tradition and the magnetic lure of the La Follette name, [Karl] enrolled at the university." Certainly Karl's mother revered Wisconsin's "Fighting Bob" La Follette, and then, too, Karl's beloved late father was born not far from Madison, in Lebanon, Wisconsin, 60 miles northeast.

2. LA PORTE

"On September 8, 1918, I came to Madison to start as an Ag College boy," Karl wrote in the notes for his memoir.

"Krish hauled my stuff," Karl wrote, referencing his younger brother, Walter, by his family nickname.

It's unclear whether the brothers traveled together or if perhaps Karl traveled by train and Walter brought his "stuff" in an automobile. In his memoir notes, Karl mentioned being "met at LaSalle Street," by "George and Pathologist," which means it was likely in Chicago, where Karl's eldest brother George received a doctorate in plant pathology in 1916 and where George would pursue a distinguished academic career. During the Chicago stop Karl changed from overalls to a suit. Next stop, college.

3. MADISON

IN MADISON, KARL WASTED little time getting himself situated. He found a clean apartment – the bottom floor of a three-story flat – at 819 West Johnson Street, just off campus. The woman renting it was a Mrs. Parker. She was asking $3 a week for the apartment.

Karl bartered, an ability he later noted he acquired as a teenager in La Porte, when he and his friend Billy Walton would sell apples in cities like Gary, South Bend and even Chicago. Billy's dad had an orchard along with the tobacco store mentioned earlier. Karl recalled taking "many a car load" of apples to Chicago and bargaining for a good price.

"I was like a skilled Armenian Oriental Rug Trader," he noted.

In Madison in September 1918, he talked Mrs. Parker down from $3 a week rent to $2.50.

Money was always going to be an issue, at least for a time. Karl's UW-Madison non-resident tuition was $52.50 for a semester; the library fee was $1 a year. Karl's brother George had encouraged him to register in Letters and Science – possibly looking toward medical school – but L & S was $20 more, so Karl chose the College of Agriculture. He nevertheless pursued science – agricultural chemistry, or what is now called biochemistry. And by his sophomore year, Karl had performed well enough in his studies to secure some scholarship funds.

Karl received a letter dated July 30, 1919 from M.E. McCaffrey, secretary of the UW Board of Regents, which stated:

3. Madison

> *"Upon the recommendation of the Faculty Committee on Loans and Undergraduate Scholarships, the Regents of the University of Wisconsin have granted you a Legislative Scholarship exempting you from the payment of non-resident tuition for the year 1919-1920."*

Still, Karl worked numerous jobs all through college. In journalist Don Behm's 1979 biographical memoir of Karl, Behm mentions a job pruning the orchard at the La Follette home in the nearby village of Maple Bluff, and quotes Karl saying, "I spent many an hour washing dishes in Sterling Court and shoveled plenty of coal in… sorority alley."

Karl's 1918 arrival in Madison coincided with the launch of a new newspaper, *The Capital Times*, published by William T. Evjue, who shared with some in the Link family an admiration for Robert M. La Follette. Karl got a job delivering and hawking the new paper. He was not warmly received at the (then) conservative University Club on campus, whose members disliked La Follette for the senator's nonintervention stand in World War I.

"Sell your damn papers somewhere else," a club member admonished Karl.

He did. Karl had an allotment of 100 papers. Sixty-five were subscribers on what was known as the "fraternity-sorority route." Karl later recalled that his customers included UW President Charles Van Hise just prior to his death, and Professor William Ellery Leonard, a poet who wrote a book about Lord Byron, which would have impressed the young Karl, who developed a keen appreciation of poetry early in his Madison stay.

Of his *Cap Times* route, Karl later recalled: "I had about 65 customers on my route, and after delivering papers to them, I would sell the balance of my 100 at corners in the campus area. I ran into tough, fighting opposition from a competing [*Wisconsin State*] *Journal* newsboy, but managed to hold my own, I believe.

"The bundle of papers would be left for me at the foot of State Street," Karl continued, "after being brought down to that point on the old streetcars. Saturdays, I would make my way to the old *Times* building on King Street to settle my weekly accounts. I gave my route over to my brother, Walter, somewhere along 1921. I made about 50 cents a day with the papers, but this helped me to get started in school and to get an education. I later had a meal job at the old Kappa Kappa Gamma House on North Park Street and secured a loan and scholarship from the late Professor Julius E. Olson.

"But it was all good training," Karl continued. "I believe I stuck it out with *The Capital Times* because I believed that it was, basically, on the right track. I needed the money, and I was an ardent admirer of the elder La Follette."

One gets a glimpse of Karl's student days in Madison in his notes for the unpublished memoir. He was "forced" to take ROTC in 1918, a circumstance made more tolerable by the enjoyment Karl took firing guns. In the notes he writes about buying, at or near age 15, a gun from a friend in La Porte. Karl would play hooky from school and walk two miles or so to a pit adjacent to a slaughterhouse where he would shoot rats "feeding on the guts of yesterday's killing." He usually got off only one shot – the rats vanished upon hearing the gunfire.

"I used to keep my gun out of sight of Mother Link," Karl noted, "who had no truck for such foolishness as shooting a rat." He would dismantle the gun walking home and keep the parts in a Pillsbury or Gold Medal flour sack.

"I doubt if I allowed myself more than 50 shots in four years," Karl noted.

In ROTC in Madison, "we were allowed to shoot with a regulation rifle – now and then."

In the memoir notes, Karl continued, "In 1918-1919 and again 1919-1920, I was given a small piece of cheap metal with a pin on it labeled Marksman 1," having scored high while firing from standing, kneeling and on-the-belly positions.

Karl recalled friends asking, "How do you do it, K.P.?"

3. MADISON

"I was not then the noisy word-spouting braggard I am now," Karl noted. His usual reply was to say his weapon was better made, or more often that the Lord had given him good eyes.

"Now and then we used to exchange guns for some control shots," Karl noted. "My performance was usually better than theirs – and so I credited 'The Lord' – and silently thanked him for my good eyes."

His ROTC shooting success was at odds with Karl's other early Wisconsin experiences. Given all he was dealing with – a new city, uncertainty about his major, difficulty with a class or two – it's not surprising Karl struggled with his emotions and moods as an undergraduate in Madison. He was hardly the first.

Freshman year, Karl's part-time work included doing odd jobs for a UW-Madison psychology professor named Joseph Jastrow. (In his memoir notes, Karl recalls the name as Jacob Jastrow, but it seems nearly certain he meant Joseph Jastrow, a Polish-American psychologist who, from 1888 until 1927, served as a professor at UW-Madison. Jastrow suffered occasional depression himself and wrote a syndicated newspaper column called "Keeping Mentally Fit.")

Karl recalled that one day he was repotting Jastrow's plants when the professor suddenly appeared through a doorway.

"Link," Jastrow said, "you're talking to yourself. What I heard indicates you are in trouble with your themes."

Karl was struggling with freshman English. His instructor was highly critical of his writing.

"A severe shock that lowered my spirits," Karl noted later, while conceding he was "at best a poor speller" unschooled in grammar and usage.

"If I flunk English," he told Jastrow, "I'm leaving this place."

The psychologist and the freshman had a long talk, during which Jastrow mentioned the subconscious – a word unfamiliar to Karl – and gave him a book on the subject. "I devoured it in one weekend – and told him that for some years I had lived exclusively on dreams, and they came out raw and unadorned in my themes."

Jastrow then introduced Karl to William Ellery Leonard, the English professor and distinguished poet whom Link knew only as a customer on his *Cap Times* paper route.

"I was too shy to speak to him," Link recalled. "I was fascinated by his eyes."

Leonard had his own issues. He suffered from agoraphobia and his first wife took her own life in 1910, a year into their marriage. Leonard later wrote an acclaimed book, "Two Lives," about the marriage.

On meeting Leonard, Link explained that Jastrow hoped Leonard might look at Karl's themes. Leonard agreed. One in particular – though marred by poor spelling – captured his interest with its unvarnished honesty. The paper was titled "I Do Not Believe in God" and dealt with Karl's father's death and "six different subjects under one heading," as Karl sheepishly noted.

Leonard, like Jastrow, encouraged Karl to keep trying, and he did. Karl managed a C in English the first quarter.

Karl worked on and off with Professor Jastrow until 1924, and at some point the professor said, "Link, I like you. Your opinions are stated in a forthright manner. You do not tell me what I would like to hear. You tell me what you think. Retain those qualities as long as you can."

Something in Karl as a young college student induced encouragement. His sophomore year, still racked with uncertainty, Karl went to see a man he identified in his memoir notes as Dr. W. S. Lorenz.

"Dr. Lorenz sized me up early," Karl noted. "Said Dr. Lorenz, 'Link, you have the temperament of a racehorse. You work too hard. You must learn to relax more.'"

Lorenz continued: "I don't think you need any drugs. But you must learn to relax. At night, just before you go to bed, take a walk – then a hot bath – and if you care to, why don't you drink a small glass of wine."

3. Madison

Lorenz concluded, "I think you should stay here – get your degree."

Karl not only got a degree, he eventually shined. The 1919 legislative scholarship mentioned earlier was the first of three and Karl was awarded membership in Phi Lambda Epsilon (an honorary chemical society) and Alpha Zeta (an honorary agricultural fraternity). In 1922, he was selected for Phi Kappa Phi, one of the nation's oldest and most selective honor societies for all academic disciplines.

On Mother's Day 1923, Karl and his brother, Walter, also enrolled at UW, sent home to Indiana a beautifully scripted poem entitled "Mother-Mine," originally written by Fairmont Snyder, the androgynous pen name of Ethel Fairmont Snyder Beebe. The poem begins: "For such as you, dear mother-mine, where worthy men, clear-eyed and frank, live by their honor code…"

Karl and Walter signed it with their family nicknames: "With love from your boys, Krish [Walter] and Chas [Karl]."

There is little question the most heartfelt and compelling record of Karl's time on the Madison campus is reflected in "Dances from Seven Years," the extraordinary leather-bound collection of oversized scrapbook pages on which Karl's hand printed prose and poetry – many of the poems are attributed to established poets – complement his photos and drawings. Paging through the first time, one might consider the book somewhat melancholy, but "searching" might be a better word. It's the product of a highly intelligent and sensitive young man beginning to find his way in the world.

There is a reverence for the beauty and mystery of nature.

"In the struggle to acquire the difficult art of living," Karl wrote in the "Fore Word," "I found my greatest friend in Nature – the trees, the waves, the winds, the shadows, the clouds, all seemed to touch me with a kindly hand.

"Some of the impressions received in my contact with nature and many of the numerous thoughts that ran through my mind while I held communion with her are reproduced here in these Dances in verse, prose and picture."

SAVING HEARTS AND KILLING RATS

Elsewhere in the foreword to what Karl calls his "booklet," he describes it as "a cycle of my life. Seven years are in it. Hard years, many times dark and lonesome, yet at the same time often extremely happy and cheerful. Therefore the mind dances, dances now here, now there, now everywhere in this booklet."

According to diaries unearthed by Katharine Coles for her 2018 book, "Look Both Ways," Karl danced for real in those early months of 1925 in Madison. He was smitten with a young woman – her name was Miriam – who was dating Karl's younger brother, Walter. Katharine Coles, Miriam, and Walter's granddaughter (Katharine's mother, Joan Link Coles, was quoted earlier in these pages), found in Miriam's diaries a passage describing meeting Karl at the Chocolate Shoppe after Miriam and Walter had seen a movie.

"K.P. and I had a battle of wits," Miriam wrote, and apparently Karl cut a dashing figure, for Walter was irritated enough to say, "She goes with the man, not the clothes."

Not long after – it was likely February 1925 – Miriam wrote that Karl "confessed his love" to her. She liked Karl – his wit and confidence – but in the end, she chose Walter, and they married. Decades later, in her book, Katharine Coles called Karl "my mother's favorite and also mine among the great aunts and uncles."

Back in 1925, Karl's dedication page for "Dances from Seven Years" read:

"To those fortunate ones – born and raised in poverty, whose early life and training has inspired them with the ideal to toil and search for the Truth – these 'Dances from Seven Years' are dedicated."

After the dedication page, Karl included a few explanatory lines, including this one: "Only a few lines of the verse are my own, the prose is mostly so."

The poets whose work Karl reproduced – in strikingly beautiful, printed script – included Poe, Longfellow, and, especially Alfred Lord Tennyson, whom Karl revered as "the greatest

3. MADISON

poet of all times – the first poet since the time of Lucretius who understood the drift of science, and whose poetical writings impress me not only as being the most profound, but at all times the most ethereal."

In an "After Note" to the booklet, Karl wrote: "Someone might ask – What do these 'Dances from Seven Years' mean? My answer is, 'How can I tell?' What does life mean? If the meaning could be given in one word, or in one picture, there would be no need of the Dances."

In closing, Karl refers – one surmises – to Tennyson, and then quotes a few lines from Tennyson's celebrated poem, "In Memoriam."

"Before a great Master, who might judge me for my past seven years I can only say –

> *"Forgive these Wild and Wandering cries*
> *"Confusions of a wasted youth*
> *"Forgive them where they toil in truth*
> *"And in thy wisdom make me wise*
>   *"for*
> *"I am but an infant crying in the night*
> *"An infant crying for the Light*
> *"And with no language but a Cry."*

At the bottom of this last page of his "Dances," Karl supplied a date: July 28, 1925.

Karl was, indeed, closing a chapter. A week earlier, on July 21, back home in La Porte, Karl had visited the clerk of court and filled out a passport application. He was planning to go to Europe.

Three years before, in June 1922, Karl received his undergraduate UW degree, a Bachelor of Science in agriculture.

"Most people," Karl wrote later, "don't know that a depression hit agriculture in the 1920s and that it was bad enough to close down agricultural implement plants and force some out of business."

Karl continued, "I had no offers of a job. No farm and no immediate prospects of finding a Home Ec. student whose parents would let me have their daughter and their farm."

In his memoir notes, Karl says he "entertained" one "wild scheme" upon graduating: "I considered going into medicine." In the end, he noted, "This would have required comparative anatomy, pathology and more physiology. That mountain looked too steep $-wise."

Instead, Karl returned to UW-Madison and got a master's degree in plant pathology in 1923. He continued to work numerous part-time jobs, one with the plant pathology department in which he counted rust spots on wheat, oats, rye and barley. It paid 30 cents an hour and the days could be long, 11 or 12 hours in the field.

Karl also worked as a waiter and laundryman at the Kappa Kappa Kappa sorority on campus and lived rent-free in an apartment house where he was responsible for collecting rents and taking care of the lawn and sidewalk.

"I came through the summer solvent," he noted, "though I sent $25 to my mother each month to help hold the house we lived in at La Porte."

That year – 1923 – Karl made his first unsuccessful application for a Rhodes Scholarship. He tried again in 1924 and finished second. That year, too, he began his Ph.D. studies under Professor William E. Tottingham.

"I was paid 40 cents an hour," Karl recalled, "for looking after his mineral absorption experiments in the green houses and I did independent work on the chemical changes that take place in the drying of plant tissues for analysis."

In 1924, presumably for a reduction in rent, Karl assumed the role of resident manager at the Bachelor Apartments, 145 Iota Court. It led to extensive correspondence with tenants and potential tenants. This was typical, from July 2, 1924:

3. MADISON

> *"Dear Mr. Link:*
>
> *"Want to confirm note that I left under your door. I rented my apartment to Mr. Ernest Kahn and advised you to that effect. I had to leave town the same day, so had little opportunity to see you personally. I am under the impression that you will collect rent for me just as long as the apartment is occupied. Wish, Mr. Link, that you would send me a copy of the lease that I signed... Very truly yours, Louis Sosland, Kansas City, Mo."*

In February 1925, as he completed his doctorate, Karl made a third and final try to secure a Rhodes Scholarship. At the completion of his oral examination, he heard one of the examiners say, "Isn't this boy a repeater?" He finished second again.

"I emerged as the alternate in the event number one conked out," Karl noted. "But number one was a jeweler's son from Milwaukee who had no intention of conking out."

Two months later, in April 1925, Karl received encouraging word from E. B. Hart, chairman of the UW Department of Agricultural Chemistry. Hart mentioned that in 1919, the Rockefeller Foundation had reached an agreement with the National Research Council to support establishing postdoctoral fellowships in physics and chemistry.

"Go see Professor Cole," Hart said.

Karl recalled "hot-footing" it to Cole's office, where he was told there was one posting for foreign study in agriculture chemistry available. An interview before the International Education Board in New York City would be required. The board would pay expenses.

On a day in May, Karl took a train to New York City. "I was too naïve to use the Pullman car," he recalled, and instead sat the entire way in coach, arriving at Grand Central Terminal at 10:00 a.m. for the 2 p.m. interview. Karl washed up in the terminal restroom and proceeded to the interview.

"I refused to sit down while questioned," Karl remembered. "This was a discipline that came from home via the late Rev. George Link."

The final question was, "Should you be selected to study abroad, what do you intend to do after?"

Karl did not hesitate. "Be a professor in agricultural chemistry somewhere."

The interview's result arrived in a letter dated June 15 and directed to E.B. Hart in Madison.

> *"My dear Professor Hart –*
>
> *"At a meeting of the International Education Board held May 29, 1925, the officers presented your nomination of Dr. Karl P. Link for a fellowship in agriculture.*
>
> *"I am happy to inform you that the Board has authorized its executive officers in their discretion to commit the Board to an appropriation to Dr. Link for a sum not to exceed $120 a month for living expenses for a period of twelve months, commencing in September 1925, and an additional sum for travel from Madison, Wisconsin to St. Andrews, Scotland, and return, to enable him to continue his studies in carbohydrate chemistry with Professor J. C. Irvine, St. Andrews University, St. Andrews, Scotland."*

Karl was headed abroad. Like so much of his life, it would prove an adventure.

4. IN SCOTLAND, SUCCESS AND CONTROVERSY

ON JULY 9, 1925, A FEW weeks after E. B. Hart received notice from the International Education Board that Karl's fellowship in Scotland was approved, J. C. Irvine, the principal at St. Andrews University, wrote Karl a letter.

> *"Dear Dr. Link,*
> *"I am very glad to learn that your appointment to an International Education Board Fellowship is now ratified and that your desire to work here can be fulfilled. A bench will be reserved for you and I shall be back in St. Andrews from vacation by the middle of September, so that you may come any day after the 15th.... You will be assured a warm welcome in the Laboratory."*

The typewritten note was hand-signed, *"Yours sincerely, J. C. Irvine."*

Karl had been interested in working with Irvine for some time, having first contacted the Scottish scientist in November 1922, just after Karl started graduate school.

Irvine wrote back on Jan. 1, 1923. "At the present moment my research laboratory is full," Irvine noted, while urging Karl to stay in touch. Karl did, and in January 1925 – even before Karl knew where money for a European trip might come from – he'd again written Irvine about working with him. Irvine responded on

Feb. 6: "The certified University record of your work at Wisconsin together with the fact that you have been since engaged in research leading to the Ph.D. Degree is quite sufficient evidence for my purpose, and I accordingly have pleasure in reserving you a place in my Research Laboratory, as from the beginning of October next."

James Colquhoun Irvine was, by 1925, on his way to being "in St. Andrews, something of a myth," in the words of his biographer, Julia Melvin.

Melvin's 2011 book, "James Colquhoun Irvine: St. Andrews' Second Founder," is an unabashedly flattering portrait of the carbohydrate chemist who in 1921 was named by the King of Scotland to the top administrative post at the University of St. Andrews, the oldest university in Scotland and the third oldest in the English-speaking world, behind Oxford and Cambridge.

Perhaps it is not surprising that the book flirts with hagiography: Melvin, the author, is Irvine's granddaughter. It is nonetheless valuable for the information it provides about Irvine, a scientist whose impact on the young Karl Paul Link was substantial.

Early in the year Irvine and Link met – 1925 – Irvine was knighted by King George V of England. He continued to run his chemistry lab even after assuming the top administrative role at St. Andrews and he was, by any measure, a formidable presence on campus and in the town.

"A man of strong passions and deep affection towards young developing minds," Melvin wrote. Later, she added: "To most of those he encountered he was a most attractive personality, but he was also strongly disliked by some of his colleagues in St. Andrews.... His autocratic command over the affairs of his alma mater was to him wise paternalism; to a few others it smacked of blind self-will."

On July 13, 1925, four days after Irvine wrote his letter welcoming Karl in advance to St. Andrews, Wallace Lund, director of fellowships for the International Education Board,

4. In Scotland, Success and Controversy

sent a note to Karl at his last Madison address (before going abroad), 145 Iota Court, in the heart of campus.

The note informed Karl that passage had been reserved for him on the SS *Montlaurier*, sailing from Quebec, Canada to Glasgow, Scotland, on August 27. Karl would be in Room 114 on board the steamer. Karl wrote back thanking Lund, noting that he would be returning to La Porte in late July and leaving for Quebec from there.

Lund in turn replied: "Your stipend for the first three months of your fellowship will be sent to you before you leave this country and will reach you at La Porte about August 10th. Your steamship ticket will also be sent about this same time." The board's assistant auditor sent Karl a check for $360 on August 5th.

By the time Karl sailed for Scotland in late August, the ship's name had been changed, to the SS *Montnairn*. Beyond that, his voyage seems to have been without incident. On September 18, Karl sent a note to Wallace Lund at the International Education Board requesting some expense reimbursement, adding that all had gone well since his arrival. Karl was lodged at a hostel called Chattan House that accommodated some two dozen male students.

"Glad to know you were so well received at St. Andrews," Lund wrote in return. "I hope that your work there is going to be exceedingly profitable."

A little less than a month later, Karl wrote Lund again from St. Andrews to say how much he was enjoying the experience – apologizing for covering ground, in his letter, not directly related to the fellowship.

Lund wrote back: "An unofficial, newsy letter of this kind needs no apology. I am always delighted to get one.

"St. Andrews is apparently an ideal place for work," Lund continued. "You mention that the only businesses in the little town are education and golf. You, of course, are devoting the major portion of your attention at the present time to education. I hope, however, that you will find plenty of time to engage in the other business of the town also." (Karl did: Among the things he saved from his time in Scotland was a local rule book for the St. Andrews Links and a pass he purchased that allowed him to play the fabled Old Course at a reduced rate.)

In his letter, Wallace Lund concluded, and this is significant: "It is gratifying to know that Principal Irvine and his associates have been so cordial to you. This will go a long way toward making your stay very enjoyable and profitable."

That letter from Lund, dated October 27, makes clear Karl and Irvine got along well at the start. So too does a note from Lund to Karl dated December 12, 1925, in response to a letter from Karl in which he stated, among other things, how much he was enjoying playing golf.

Lund pronounced himself "very pleased that you have taken the time to write such a newsy informal letter.... Other fellows will perhaps be going to St. Andrews and will want to know in advance what may be expected there in the way of equipment, golf, etc. I am interested to know that you have taken such an interest in golf. This is a fine recreation and if you do not take it too seriously should go far to relieve the tension occasioned by your intensive studies and research."

Karl was enjoying his experience overseas so much that in a Christmas 1925 note home to E. B. Hart in Madison, he stated the hope his fellowship might be extended beyond early 1927, when he was expected back at UW-Madison. (Once his year at St. Andrews was up, Karl had visits planned to the laboratories of the eminent scientists Hans Pringsheim in Berlin, Fritz Pregl in Austria, and Paul Karrer in Switzerland. This required a six-month extension of his fellowship, but as noted, Karl was hoping for an extension.)

Hart and the Agricultural Chemistry Department had offered Karl an assistant professorship at a salary of $3,000, which included a summer appointment, with a start date of February 1, 1927.

4. In Scotland, Success and Controversy

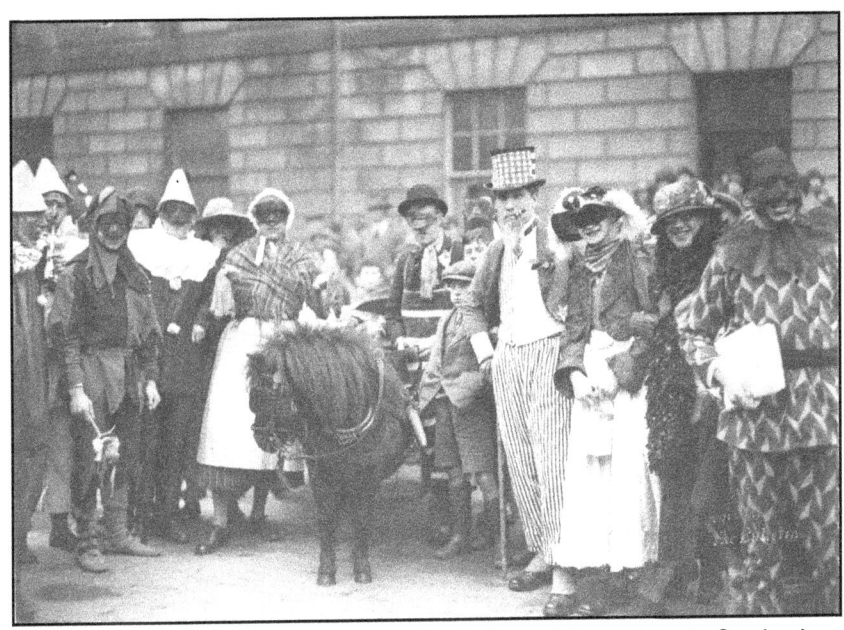

Karl, often a showman, dressed as Uncle Sam while studying in Scotland.
(Link family)

Hart responded to Karl's Christmas letter on January 19, 1926. Hart's response has a friendly, encouraging tone, but it's evident Hart and the leadership of the department of plant pathology in Madison did not want Karl to stay too long in Europe.

"I took up your proposal of staying another year with the plant people (Professors Jones, Dickson, and Tottingham)," Hart wrote, "and while they all appreciate your point of view, they felt that the lapse of two years without contact with their program would be too long a delay...."

"I believe that your future here has great prospects," Hart continued. "The men in plant lines are interested in making this one of two or three leading centers in the country for plant chemistry and I believe that your association with that work would add materially to its progress was well as establish a reputation for yourself."

Hart said he looked forward to Karl starting February 1, 1927.

At the same time – January 1926 – Karl heard from James Dickson, a UW-Madison associate professor of plant pathology. Karl had sent Dickson reports of his research with Irvine on cellulose – the substance that makes up most of a plant's cell walls. Much of Dickson's January 20 letter is of a highly scientific nature regarding cell walls and microchemical reactions. But Dickson, too, urged Karl to return to Madison for the start of the spring semester in February 1927.

"Professor Jones and I have talked this over," Dickson wrote, "and we are rather inclined to suggest that you so plan your work as to reach Madison somewhere about February 1."

Karl agreed, sending a note in early February 1926 to Hart in Madison saying he planned to be back for the spring 1927 semester (commencing February 1). In hindsight, this may have been an early crack in Karl's relationship with Irvine. The St. Andrews principal and scientific researcher did not want Karl to leave Scotland in the middle of an investigation.

On February 25, 1926, Irvine wrote a letter to E. B. Hart in Madison, expressing his concern and wish that Karl prolong his stay.

On March 13, Hart responded.

"My dear Dr. Irvine: I have your letter and am very glad to know of the distinct progress you are making on the constitution of cellulose and that Dr. Link is taking a part in that work.

"I appreciate fully your point of view that it is highly disadvantageous to break off a piece of research at a point where there is a possibility of loss to the investigator whether it be in credit or results."

That said, Hart continued, Wisconsin wanted Karl back. Jones and Dickson in plant pathology, Hart wrote, "feel that he should make his plans to be back with us February 1, 1927. We already have him in our budget for next year...."

Within three months of this exchange – by mid-June 1926 – something happened that completely soured the relationship

4. In Scottland, Success and Controversy

between Irvine and Karl. Whatever it was, it was serious. Karl left St. Andrews abruptly. And no matter Karl's promising potential as a young scientist, such a break – a falling out with an elder as prominent as Irvine – threatened to sidetrack Karl's nascent career.

"Link's version," wrote Robert H. Burris, years later, "was that he made an observation in conflict with a concept of Irvine, and because he refused to compromise his principles, he was asked to leave."

On June 15, Ettie Steel, who began at St. Andrews as a research chemist but by 1926 was Irvine's personal secretary, wrote Karl a note on university stationery.

"Dear Dr. Link: I am sorry to trouble you when you are 'on the move,' but your report cannot be found anywhere. The Principal is anxious to get hold of it and would be very grateful if you would drop him a card to say where it may be found. I'm sorry I didn't see you to say goodbye, so allow me to wish you a good time while you are on your travels and good luck in the future."

Karl's reply, dated June 23, was curt.

"Dear Dr. Steele: The report of the work I did under Professor Irvine's direction will be sent to him as soon as I have it written. I should like to state that I had told Principal Irvine explicitly that the report was not written on Saturday June 13 and that it would be sent to him when it was completed."

A second letter sent to Link, a day after Ettie Steel's, came from a man Karl called "the laboratory detective," and it was far less genial, asking that Karl return lab materials "if they have been removed by you. If they have been left in the laboratory, will you please inform me where they are."

In notes handwritten on this typed letter, Karl remarked that he had told Irvine that he would put all materials in a "compartment of my desk – which of course I did."

Karl's leaving St. Andrews did not end the rift. Irvine stated his intention to file a complaint against Karl with the Standing

Committee of Vice Chancellors of the Universities of Great Britain, in hopes Karl would be prevented in the future from entering any university in the British Empire. He wrote a similarly venomous letter to Wickliffe Rose, president of the International Education Board. And he contacted Hans Pringsheim in Germany, urging the scientist to disinvite Karl, who was expected in Pringsheim's lab in Berlin in the fall.

Pringsheim immediately sent a note to a secretary at St. Andrews: "I beg you to inform Dr. Karl Paul Link that according to a change in my dispositions I shall not be able to have him work with me in Berlin."

Burris, in his biograph of Karl, wrote: "The incident caused such a hassle that in a subsequent year when Elizabeth McCoy's application was being considered for a comparable fellowship, the question was raised whether the board could risk having another University of Wisconsin appointee."

It is important to note that Karl did not back down. He was 25 years old, in a foreign country, his integrity under assault by the most esteemed man at the third oldest English-speaking university in the world – and he did not back down.

By mid-July, Karl had rearranged his schedule. It now called for him to make a stop in Paris at the Institut Pasteur, followed by six weeks in the laboratory of Fritz Pregl in Graz, Austria, finishing in the lab of Paul Karrer in Zurich, Switzerland.

Karl was also writing letters, explaining what had happened at St. Andrews, telling his side of the story.

He was aided in this by a correspondence with W. Norman Haworth, who in 1925 was director of the chemistry department at the University of Birmingham. Haworth was already an esteemed scientist, and in 1937, a dozen years after his correspondence with Karl, he would win the Nobel Prize in Chemistry for his work with carbohydrates and vitamin C.

A friend at St. Andrews told Karl that Haworth had experienced a similar disintegration of his relationship with Irvine at St. Andrews, where Haworth arrived as a lecturer in 1912.

4. IN SCOTLAND, SUCCESS AND CONTROVERSY

In Julia Melvin's biography of Irvine, she wrote, without documenting the source of the discord, that Haworth left St. Andrews in 1920 after "a blazing row" with Irvine.

When Karl reached out to Haworth, the older scientist responded in a manner that must have heartened Karl. The letter does not survive, but Karl shared it with colleagues at UW-Madison, and one, Professor R. A. Brink in the Department of Genetics, wrote Karl: "Haworth's letter produced a great impression here and did a great deal to offset Irvine's incriminating and slanderous statements."

In mid-July, about a month after Karl left St. Andrews, he received a calming letter from E. B. Hart, the professor in Madison who first told him about the chance for an overseas fellowship.

"I received your London letter today detailing your controversy with Dr. Irvine," Hart wrote on July 13.

Hart noted that Irvine had also been in touch, denouncing Karl and enclosing the letter he, Irvine, wrote to Wickliffe Rose at the International Education Board.

"We have confidence in you back here," Hart wrote. "I talked the matter over with [Professor James] Dickson the other day and, as one of us said, it looks like a scrap between a Scotchman and a German, and we will let it go at that."

Hart continued, "If Dr. Irvine is exploiting his students as you say he is, then, of course, the axe falls on him and not on you.... A rumpus with another fellow – if that rumpus is based on good faith and a defense of ethical principles – isn't going to deter the University of Wisconsin from employing you and giving you a chance for scientific development."

Karl, in his letter, must have expressed at least some apprehension about his future, because Hart added, "Don't be so youthful as to want to give up your science, because that is wholly unnecessary."

Karl's most complete and passionate explanation of the controversy came in an undated – though it must have been summer 1926 – handwritten letter to Claude Burton Hutchinson, the American, Paris-based International Education Board's director for Europe. Given its gravitas, the letter deserves quoting at some length, though in places Karl's handwriting is hard to decipher. The bracketed words represent the author's best interpretation of the handwriting.

"My dear Prof. Hutchinson," Karl wrote. "The experience I had working at St. Andrews under Principal J. C. Irvine has proven to be a very unhappy, unsatisfactory and unfortunate one. Things did not go well from the start but I tried to be happy.... Rather foolishly I did not complain to any official of the International Education Board. In fact my letters to the Wisconsin men who were responsible for getting me the fellowship never [explained] the situation I was in. The unfortunate position was hidden behind a screen of optimism. To overcome my disappointment I worked like a Trojan on a [project] of my own along with the work Irvine had started me on.

"It is," Karl continued, "perhaps a characteristic of youth to be a little too credulous and to hold an overrated and [unearned] respect for British men of the rank of Mr. Irvine, who have been knighted, etc., etc. [Interestingly] I saw through Mr. Irvine's methods almost at once. However I did not permit myself to be guided by my [intuitive] sense. I tried to make myself believe I liked the man and his system. Toward the end actual experience and [regular] contact with him brought me to the conclusions I had known intuitively."

Karl's concluding paragraph was especially heartfelt.

"My experience needs to be told, Mr. Hutchinson," Karl wrote. "It cannot be written in a few words. I can tell you how I found Mr. Irvine. He is one of the cleverest and canny men I have ever seen – but not honest (Karl underlined the words 'but not honest' three times). His whole career is [filled] with students, colleagues and coworkers whom he has exploited and trampled on all for his own fame and glory. When he tried to exploit me – I

4. In Scottland, Success and Controversy

challenged him. His policy is to get as much as you can from the man around you, give him nothing, yet have him think he is getting something. A more clever scientific bluffer I would never hope to see."

No, Karl did not back down.

He and Hutchinson spoke by phone on July 15 and 16. Whether Karl elaborated on the points he made in the undated letter is not clear, but in two written responses dated July 16 – sent to Karl in Paris – Hutchinson expressed no qualms about Karl continuing his European fellowship. It is possible the International Education Board briefly suspended his fellowship – Karl alludes to that happening in his unpublished memoir. But Hutchinson – who later in life served as mayor of Berkeley, California – authorized payment for Karl's revised itinerary, which now included visits with Professor Bertrand at the Institut Pasteur and Professor Fernbach at the Brewers Institute, both in Paris, a total of 10 days; a stop of several days in Heidelberg with Professor Freudenberg; followed by several days with Professor Paul Karrer in Zurich; then six weeks in Graz, Austria with Professor Fritz Pregl; and, last, an extended stay returning to the lab of either Freudenberg in Germany or Karrer in Switzerland (Karl chose Karrer). The fellowship, Hutchinson reminded Karl, "terminates about the end of January, 1927."

Throughout the summer and fall of 1926, Karl continued to receive correspondence related to the Irvine controversy.

Karl had written, asking for support, to D'Arcy Wentworth Thompson, a large presence at St. Andrews, nearly the equal of Irvine. Thompson – later knighted – was a founder of mathematical biology who in 1917 became chairman of natural history at St. Andrews University.

He was not completely unsympathetic to Karl, but neither was he willing to speak for him publicly.

"My dear Boy," Thompson wrote in an August 16 letter, when Karl was in Zurich, on his first visit with Paul Karrer. "You must not and cannot expect me to help you; to do so, or to espouse your cause in any way, or even to enquire into the rights and wrongs of this unhappy affair, it is beyond my powers. You have quarreled with a man whom we all know to be an unflinching opponent, a bitter enemy if you prefer the words."

Thompson concluded, "You are probably seeing Karrer now, while I am writing you. I do hope you will find him helpful, and that with his help you may find a way out of your troubles. Many if not most of these are of your own making, that I am sure of, but I am not without sympathy for you on that account."

Karl's family back in the United States was kept current on his situation. Karl's sister Ruth sent a $1,000 loan when his St. Andrews stay was abruptly terminated. And it was an August 20 letter from a family member – Karl's sister-in-law, Adeline, wife of his eldest brother, George – that may have come closest to articulating the root cause of the controversy.

"I dope out the situation as follows," Adeline wrote. "(You have never really told us just what is the crux of the matter, so I have to reconstruct it from reading between the lines, so I may be wide of the mark.) I judge that the 'last straw' was probably a cool assumption on the part of Irvine that results which you had obtained through your own independent efforts be published as the product of Irvine and Link. Am I right? Of course that was merely 'the straw that broke the camel's back,' but my hunch is that something like that came as the climax of a series of indignities against which you had been chafing.

"At any rate," Adeline theorized, "whatever the immediate cause, you, with just cause, 'blew up,' and probably told Irvine quite truthfully and possibly accurately, just what he is! Whereupon he in turn exploded more violently and the row was on."

In mid-September 1926, three months after the Irvine controversy ignited, E. B. Hart wrote Karl from Madison, encouraging him to move beyond it. (Hart had said as much in a previous letter in mid-July.)

"I think you should drop this whole matter of Irvine and devote your time and your thoughts to your work," Hart wrote.

4. In Scottland, Success and Controversy

"Your time in Europe is limited and you should make the most of your time for your own advancement. It will gain you nothing to attempt to put up a case against Irvine except to keep you stirred up and your mind away from your work… The future will decide Irvine's place and the important thing for you is to profit from your stay in Europe…. Now take my advice and drop the whole thing and go ahead with your work because, in the long run, I have never seen very many people stay interested in a controversy. I am mighty glad you are enjoying your work on micro analysis and I hope you will have a fine stay in Zurich."

Karl did move past it. In September 1927 – just before returning to the United States from Europe – he wrote Irvine a letter saying, as Karl later paraphrased it, "that whilst I most likely could never wipe that raw-deal from my mind, I was ready to forgive his error."

In his unpublished memoir, Karl wrote briefly about the subsequent contact he had with Irvine.

"I had a couple of letters from him between 1927 and 1937," Karl wrote. "Then I heard nothing until 1946, upon the occasion of my election to the National Academy of Sciences. J. C. Irvine was a foreign member, and he was decent enough to write me when he learned that I was elected to the Academy."

Karl continued, "He also told me about his troubles – the loss of his only son [who had drowned]. I remember the boy – he used to collect all the American stamps from my letters."

Over time, Karl also stayed in touch with another figure at St. Andrews, D'Arcy Wentworth Thompson, who had declined to support Karl during his falling out with Irvine. Or at least Karl made a point of letting Thompson know about the breakthrough he made with dicumarol.

On Jan. 1, 1945, Thompson wrote Karl a note in response: "You are by no means forgotten here, and it was a pleasure to hear from you. But you might let us have a little more news of your doings than is contained in a paper on Sweet Clover Hay!"

Saving Hearts and Killing Rats

After St. Andrews, the next part of Karl's 1925-27 European adventure went much better. In September 1926, after a brief stop with Paul Karrer in Zurich – where he would return for a lengthier stay – Karl landed in Graz, Austria, 90 miles south of Vienna, and began a rewarding association with Fritz Pregl, the Austrian chemist who won the Nobel Prize in 1923 for his work with microanalysis. Pregl ran the Institute for Medical Chemistry at the University of Graz.

Karl liked and admired Pregl, sentiments, we will see, that were returned by the older scientist.

"Pregl had developed microchemistry to a fine art," wrote Robert Burris in his biograph of Karl, "and Link was fascinated by the techniques and mastered them."

In his biographical memoir of Karl, journalist Don Behm stressed the personal connection.

"Karl Paul gained Pregl's personal attention at Graz," Behm wrote, "and was invited to an evening assembly where many of the unusual names for microtools (such as *Dachhundbrenner*) were created. Pregl also invited K.P.L. to the famous *Herringsalat* [herring salad] on Ash Wednesday, a special ceremony usually reserved for Pregl's closest European friends."

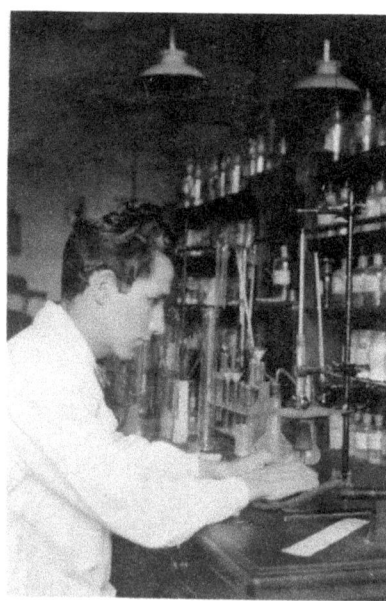

Karl in Graz, Austria, in 1926, where he was studying with the distinguished scientist Fritz Pregl, winner of the Nobel Prize for Chemistry. (Link family)

4. In Scotland, Success and Controversy

UW-Madison biochemist Dave Nelson, whose keen insights into Karl's life and work are always helpful, calls Karl's time with Pregl "one of the most important things he did" as a young scientist.

"Pregl at that time," Nelson said, "was in the process of winning the Nobel Prize for his development of techniques for microanalysis – techniques that allowed one to look at very small quantities of a chemical compound and to determine its composition and therefore its identity.

"While Link was in Pregl's lab," Nelson continued, "he learned those techniques."

According to Nelson, Karl brought back a piece of microanalytical equipment that may have been the first of its kind on this side of the Atlantic. (It is now housed in the Wisconsin State Historical Society Museum.)

"In those days," Nelson continued, "it allowed a scientist to isolate a compound from nature, to determine its composition and structure, and in some cases to improve on its structure by chemical synthesis and make another compound that might have the same or stronger effect. That's where Link began."

Karl and Pregl were close enough that they stayed in touch after Karl returned to the United States in summer 1927. One letter survives, written by Pregl to Karl in Madison in May 1929 in response to one from Karl.

It's likely that Karl's mastery of the German language enhanced his relationship with Pregl, particularly in the early going, and Pregl's letter to Karl was written in German. What follows is the English translation:

"Many thanks for your long letter," Pregl wrote, "from which I gather that the seeds planted here in my Institute have successfully born fruit in America and that you are using microanalysis as an indispensable resource in your scientific work, and that you will disseminate it further among your students. I congratulate you on your scientific successes and your promotion to Associate Professor.

"I will gladly fulfill your request for a photograph, which is being mailed to you at the same time as this letter, carefully packed.

"The fact that you recall the amusing times from your stay in Graz, such as the herring salad and similar things, I count among your good qualities.

"Heartfelt greetings from all members of the Institute, and from, yours sincerely,

"Prof. Fritz Pregl."

Two small photographs of Pregl are with Karl's papers in the University of Wisconsin Archives.

Karl's admiration for Pregl was further revealed when Pregl died in December 1930 after contracting pneumonia. He was 61. Karl immediately formulated a plan to give a memorial lecture in Pregl's honor. It would be in the Agricultural Chemistry Building on the UW-Madison campus at 8 p.m. on March 13, 1931.

Karl had his personal experience to draw on for the lecture, and he also reached out to people like Oskar Wintersteiner, a professor of biochemistry at Columbia University in New York City. Wintersteiner was a native of Austria who studied under Pregl at the University of Graz, earning a doctorate in 1921, five years before Karl's arrival. (Karl and Wintersteiner just missed each other in Graz; earlier in 1926, prior to Karl's arrival, Wintersteiner left for an International Education Board fellowship in the United States at Johns Hopkins.)

In February 1931, Wintersteiner responded from New York to Karl's request for information on Pregl for his memorial lecture. The following paragraph from Wintersteiner's letter is interesting in that his description of Pregl's personality and working method seem in accordance with Karl's own. Maybe it's not surprising the two got on so well.

"Pregl's method of working out a problem," Wintersteiner wrote Karl, "reflected very much his impetuous personality and intuitive type of mind. If he once became involved with a prob-

4. In Scotland, Success and Controversy

lem, he devoted all his time and ruthless energy to bringing it to a satisfactory solution, working day and night at it with an almost superhuman intensity until it was solved, and then he relaxed into a period of comparative inertia which lasted until a new problem approached him closely enough to incense his imagination."

On March 4, 1931, Karl sent a letter to Dr. Walter Meek, assistant dean of medicine at the University of Wisconsin Medical School, noting how Pregl's studies as a medical student in Innsbruck and Graz had prepared him for an illustrious career.

"If you would be so kind as to announce this lecture to those medical students who might be interested I would be very grateful to you," Karl wrote, adding that "all of the apparatuses designed and devised by Pregl will be on display."

Karl's talk that night in Madison is notable for the window it provides into his own views on chemistry.

"Chemistry is both a craft and an art," Karl began. "It is at one and the same time one of the finest crafts and one of the finest arts, perhaps the art of arts, a veritable sword wherewith the threads are cut which hold the secrets of our material world and the nature and character of its component units. It has a wondrous psychology of which but a few as yet have gained feeling, mastery and reverence.

"Chemistry is with respect to mathematics and physics a science only in the second degree," Karl continued, "because of so much of its burden cannot be quantified. It is, nevertheless, a premier science, through the exquisite finish of the enviable craftsmanship exercised by the men of genius who have been successful in its service.

"Among the craftsmen who have most adorned our ranks we can place none higher than the one to whom this evening is dedicated, for he had reached the highest pinnacle of technical proficiency to which our art is carried. A striking feature in his conquests has been the sureness and swiftness of his approach, the courage of his outlook and his deft handling of situations which previous workers had failed to master."

Later in his lecture, describing Pregl's microanalytical breakthrough, Karl said, "He finally, at the age of 41, in the course of a lengthy physiological investigation reached a climax which brought him face to face with the existing development in organic analysis. A big idea came to him; he set out to extend the boundaries of analysis. This idea to create accurate microanalysis methods ruled him and forced him through a hell and heaven."

The phrase going through "a hell and heaven" might also serve as an apt epitaph for Karl's 1925-1927 European fellowship. The nightmare of his stay with Irvine in St. Andrews was outweighed, finally, by his rewarding work and friendship with Pregl.

Karl's last months in Europe might best be described as anticlimactic. He was working under Paul Karrer at the Chemical Institute at the University of Zurich in Switzerland, and while Karrer was a brilliant scientist – he would win the Nobel in 1937 for his research on vitamins – Karrer's work was not closely related to the carbohydrate chemistry that excited Karl. It might be coincidence, but at this time Karl began to dress with a certain flair – knickers, a cape, he even grew a beard.

He also suffered a flare-up of the tuberculosis Karl occasionally claimed he had first contracted as a very young boy.

"He spent weekends at a tuberculosis retreat in Davos," wrote Burris in his biograph of Karl.

"He was threatened with tuberculosis," Behm wrote, "and required to spend each weekend from November through March at Davos, a tuberculosis retreat in the Swiss Alps."

Nevertheless, Karl hoped to extend his stay in Europe until fall 1927, when he planned to return to his teaching position at UW-Madison. He applied for a fellowship extension.

In mid-February 1927, Karl received a letter in Zurich from E. B. Hart in Madison. Hart notes that Karl's colleagues in agricultural chemistry at UW had written the International Education Board "endorsing an extension of your [fellowship]. I hope you get it, although it is rather late to be making the request.

4. In Scottland, Success and Controversy

I presume you have already done it, but you should certainly have Dr. Karrer write the Board for you... I am very glad to know you are getting along well and that you will be back with us in the fall."

The following month, Karl received a letter from C. B. Hutchinson, the board's director for Europe, whom he got to know during the Irvine controversy.

"The board has found it impractical to grant your request for a second extension of your fellowship for a period of six months," Hutchinson wrote on March 18. "Regretting the disappointment this letter will bring you."

One last anecdote from Zurich is worth noting. Years later, Karl recalled it in a wry note to a friend.

"It is perhaps somewhat ironic," Karl wrote, "that among my personal possessions – in German script – is a scrap of paper with the words: 'Karl Paul Gerhard Link, anno Domini [in the year of the Lord] 1/31/1901, What manner of child shall this be: Luke 1:66.'

"I found this many years ago," Karl continued, "in my father's Lutheran hymnal. I got a terrific shock in 1926, while a student in Zurich, Switzerland, where a professor of philosophy – in a discourse on Nietzsche – indicated that Nietzsche's father inserted in the church register in Rocken at Friedrich's christening the same lines from Luke."

Karl said he was momentarily pleased to share this connection with Nietzsche, but added: "In January 1889, according to this professor, Nietzsche went hopelessly mad."

Even without the fellowship funds, Karl stayed in Europe until June. He sailed for New York from Bremen, Germany, on June 23, 1927, aboard the SS *Columbus*, and moved back in briefly to the family home in La Porte, Indiana.

On July 15, E. B. Hart – the chairman of the agricultural chemistry department and Karl's main contact in Madison – wrote Karl a letter in La Porte, in response to a letter in which Karl noted he'd arrived in the United States absent both his beard and his golf clubs.

"You should have kept your whiskers," Hart wrote. "I think it would have been great fun to have you roll into Madison with whiskers.

"I am sorry you lost your clubs," Hart continued, "because you will have to get a new set to keep in touch with the bunch around here. We have a municipal course now and they are all playing golf whenever they get a little time."

Getting to business, Hart added, "I have told some of the members of the Chemistry Conference that you were to be the carbohydrate chemist on the campus and I hope that is final... Let me add that the salary of $2,400 that I have put in is for the academic year, and summer pay for station workers carries one-eighth of that salary in addition."

A decades-long career on the UW-Madison campus was at hand.

5. ELIZABETH

ONCE BACK IN MADISON, Karl hit the ground running. He'd brought back from Europe not only his training from Pregl on determining the structure of carbohydrates, but a device he'd worked with that allowed for the analysis of very small quantities of organic material.

"There were two parts to the device," Dave Nelson said – an analytical balance that could weigh miniscule quantities, and what was called a combustion train, which analyzed a compound as it moved through. In the end one could determine the percentages of carbon, nitrogen and oxygen present in the material. The device help jumpstart Karl's research and got people's attention.

"Link returned to an assistant professorship in agricultural chemistry," Burris wrote in his biograph. "In 1928 he was promoted to associate professor. The staff knew K. P. Link was capable as a teacher and researcher, and he justified their confidence many times over."

"His laboratory work," Don Behm wrote of the same 1927-1928 period, "included the identification of Hexuronic Acids, the biochemistry of diseases resistant to plants, and the isolation of Protocatechuic Acid from pigmented onion scales. Protocatechuic Acid is the chemical compound that enables colored onions to resist smudge diseases."

In December 1928, E. B. Hart sent a manuscript to Dr. D. D. Van Slyke, who was on the editorial board of the *Journal of Biological Chemistry* and based at the Rockefeller Institute for Medical Research in New York City.

"My dear Dr. Van Slyke:

"We are sending you today," Hart wrote in a cover note, "a manuscript by Dr. Link and associates, dealing with the 'Isolation of Protocatechuic Acid from Pigmented Onion Scales' and the significance of this isolation. While I am aware that the Journal has not leaned very heavily toward plant chemical research, I think this paper is so distinctive and pioneering in its character that it should find a place in a high grade biochemical journal. For that reason I hope that it will be given careful consideration by your Committee and be published in due time in the *Journal of Biological Chemistry*."

In fact, the journal published it almost immediately, in 1929, under the title "The Isolation of Protocatechuic Acid from Pigmented Onions and Its Significance in Relation to Disease Resistance in Onions."

Karl's star was in ascendance. Early on, he had caught the eye of C. S. Slichter, a mathematics professor and subsequently dean of the graduate school at UW-Madison. As a freshman, Karl took Slichter's agricultural mathematics course and he later recalled how the professor enjoyed Karl's correctly answering a question from his understanding of plowing, not math. For his part, Karl liked Slichter's approach to teaching, which he described as, "I'm going to try to make mathematics easy for you, and interesting."

The two stayed in touch while Karl was in graduate school, and after his return to Madison from Europe. The extent to which Slichter championed Karl can be seen in a Dec. 10, 1930 letter written by Slichter to Thomas Brittingham, Jr., the public face of UW-Madison's Brittingham Fund, which had been established in the wills of Brittingham's parents. (Thomas Jr., in 1925, was one of the founders of the Wisconsin Alumni Research Foundation, or WARF, which would eventually play an important role in Karl's life.)

Slichter wrote Brittingham suggesting that the fund underwrite a five-year appointment for Karl – a "Brittingham Research

5. ELIZABETH

Professorship in Bio-Chemistry." The amount of money proposed – $27,500 for the five years – would nearly double Karl's current salary of around $3,000 annually.

"In explanation of this suggestion," Slichter wrote, "I will state that there has been under way in various laboratories of the University of Wisconsin for a number of years a study of a group of fundamental problems in the Chemistry of Vital Processes in which results of great scientific importance have already been obtained and which we are very desirous of developing further in the future. The work of Mr. Link forms an important part of that program...

"Mr. Link's work has been especially associated with what we may call plant chemistry," Slichter continued. "During the last year he has printed seven papers having to do with the phenomena of the production of organic compounds in the living plant. A strong combination of interest in all the allied problems in the fields of both plant and animal physiology, bio-chemistry, experimental zoology, and plant pathology already exists and is of long standing and has drawn the departments into active cooperation. It is obvious that this cooperation can not be forced but must take place in the natural course of events by the similarity of the ends sought and by the enthusiasms of the various research workers.

"Mr. Link is a young man well trained abroad in organic and bio-chemistry. He has studied at St. Andrews in Scotland, in Switzerland and in Vienna. As far as it is possible to predict human affairs, we believe it is safe to appoint him to this position of honor and to be reasonably certain that his five years of research will be both productive and of a character materially to advance this important field of science and that the results will be of satisfaction to the donors of the fund."

The Brittingham Fund responded positively. It was not, however, without controversy, a point of discord between the university and the Brittingham trust that goes unmentioned in the biographical memoirs of Karl by Don Behm and Robert Burris.

Burris does not mention the Brittingham fund at all, while Behm notes:

"The [Brittingham] trustees accepted the proposal, appointing Karl Paul the first Professor of Biochemistry at Wisconsin in 1930."

It appears Behm was in error on the year: It was at a March 1931 meeting of the executive committee of the UW Board of Regents that Karl's five-year appointment was approved, "the funds for Professor Link's salary to be provided by the Brittingham University of Wisconsin Trust."

In the end, it wasn't that simple. A series of articles in *The Capital Times* questioned whether a private fund should be dictating how university money is spent. The debate grew heated. It seems an early example of Karl being a lightning rod for controversy even in circumstances not of his own making.

The top page one headline in the June 20, 1931 *Capital Times* read: "Regents Refuse Brittingham Funds." The secondary headline read: "Turn Down Money for Link Pay."

The story began, "University regents today rejected all funds paid by the Brittingham estate to the university for the salary of Karl Paul Link as Brittingham professor of biochemistry... By this action, the regents expressed their intention of not permitting trustees of the Brittingham estate to dictate whose salary the trust fund should pay at the university... Prof. Link will continue on the university payroll, paid by university funds."

The last mention of the controversy in a Madison newspaper came three months later, on Sept. 23 in *The Capital Times*, a short story on an inside page headlined, "'Tainted Funds' Question Still Faces U.W."

The Cap Times noted: "Because Mr. [Thomas] Brittingham sought to dictate terms of the Link appointment, the regents rebelled..."

"The situation remains cloudy," the paper concluded, "with the university policy pretty much undecided."

5. ELIZABETH

It probably was not of critical importance to Karl, who after all was getting paid one way or another. It does appear that the Brittingham funds were finally made available to subsidize Karl, or at least one gleans as much from a 1942 lecture Karl gave to the Madison Literary Club, in which he credits the Brittingham funds for helping him establish a first-rate lab.

In any case, as was true throughout his life, one never wanted to be too certain about what would spark Karl's interest or ire. Often it had to do with a perceived misuse of authority. In those cases, there was little question which side Karl would be on.

A year earlier, in spring 1930, a German shepherd police dog that also served as the mascot of a UW fraternity, Sigma Nu, was shot dead for "trespassing" on the property of a wealthy lumberman, E. J. Young, who owned Picnic Point. It caused a brief uproar in Madison. *The Daily Cardinal* student newspaper editorialized in support of the dog, named Franz, and noted, "We hope that dog heaven is a pleasant place of fields without fences. In that land beyond the sky there should be some kindness since there is so little of it here."

The *Cardinal* suggested a memorial stone in honor of Franz, to be inscribed, "Erected by students and townspeople of Madison who still make a distinction between wealth and omnipotence."

Two days later, *The Capital Times* published a list of "fourteen new contributors" to a fund to erect the monument honoring Franz. Among the names: Prof. Karl Paul Link.

That year – 1930 – was of surpassing importance in Karl's personal life. According to Don Behm, he cut a dashing figure on returning from Europe, often wearing a cape, and woolen knickers with red fringes. Karl's archive contains some correspondence from women while he was abroad, including an early 1926 letter from Wilma Ott of Chicago, who most likely met Karl on the Madison campus.

She wrote Karl in Scotland after receiving his 1925 Christmas card from St. Andrews. It's a warm letter, and concludes,

"Hope I'll hear from you again, Karl. I've often wished last summer had been a little longer. At any rate, remember my very best wishes are with you."

It was almost exactly a year after Karl's return to the United States in summer 1927 that he had a date that changed his life. On July 4, 1928, Karl rented a canoe from the University of Wisconsin boathouse on Lake Mendota, behind the Red Gym, and rowed a young woman friend out to Picnic Point. A student friend of Karl's named Bill Olson had introduced them. The young woman's name was Elizabeth Feldman and as the story was passed down in the family, Karl and Elizabeth – Lisa – stayed out so long that her mother phoned the boathouse numerous times, increasingly concerned, to see if they had returned.

"I fell in love on July 4, 1928," Karl wrote, two decades later, "and never got over it."

Elizabeth was part of a distinguished Madison family. Her mother Molly Kailin's family was one of the first Jewish families

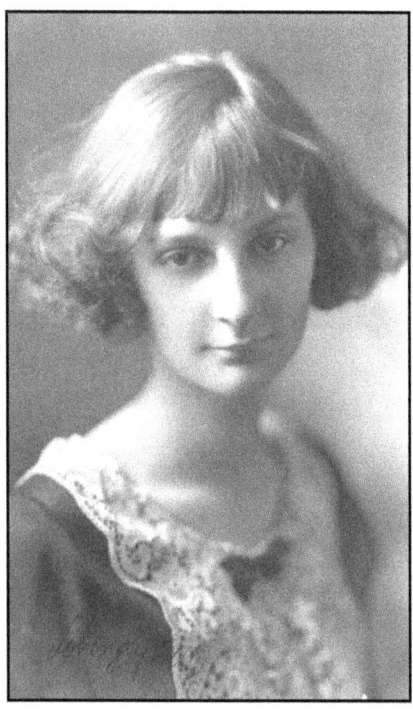

Elizabeth Feldman, prior to meeting Karl. (Link family)

5. Elizabeth

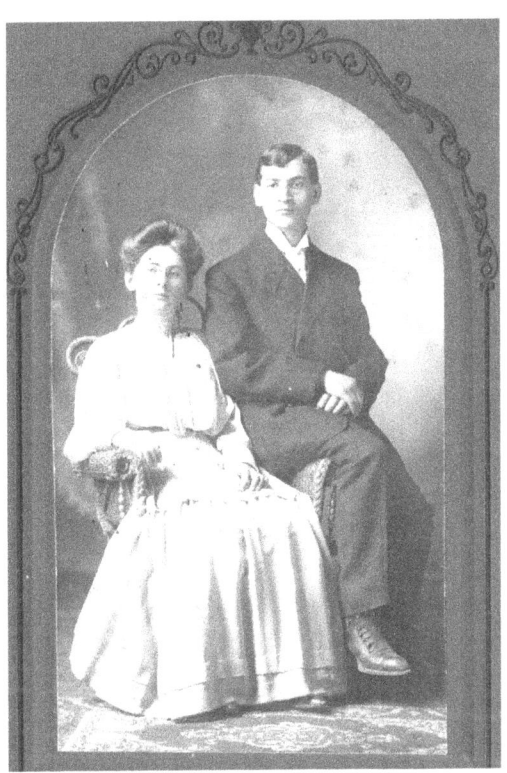

Molly Kailin Feldman and Jacob Feldman, Elizabeth's parents. (Link family)

to settle in Madison, having immigrated to Wisconsin from Minsk, Russia a few years after Molly's birth in 1884.

Her father, Jacob Feldman, had an extraordinary early life. He was born in Warsaw, Poland, in 1888, one of seven children of a road contractor who worked for the Russian government. Jacob attended Jewish parochial schools and was studying to be a rabbi when, at age 13, he changed course. He got a job at a stationery factory, earning three rubles – or $1.50 – a month. It led to a job with increased responsibility at a box factory, an experience Jacob would draw on later, after immigrating to the United States.

That move was precipitated after Jacob was among a group of young people arrested at a meeting that authorities rightly believed was subversive in nature. It was 1904; a revolution against the tyrannical Russian autocracy was at hand. Jacob was jailed, held for several months – he later recalled being allowed five minutes daily for exercise – and upon his release paid a smuggler to get him covertly to Prussia. There he was able to contact his father, who had already crossed to the United States, settling in Wisconsin. His father sent passage money and Jacob joined him in Madison. It was spring 1905.

"In a year he could read, write and speak the language," according to a profile of Jacob Feldman that appeared years later in *The Capital Times*.

He had ambition and drive. Jacob used his Warsaw experience to land a job with Madison's Democrat Printing Company and saved enough money in a couple of years to buy a small grocery store. In 1909, he sold that and purchased a larger store at the corner of Randall and University Avenue in Madison. (Jacob and his family would live in an apartment above the grocery store.) His goal was a box factory, the business he'd learned before fleeing Poland. Toward that end he bought property in 1914 at 29 North Charter Street. But it wasn't until 1921 that Jacob sold the grocery store and started the Feldman Paper Box Company at the Charter Street location. Within a decade, it employed 125 people in peak season with annual revenues of $70,000.

Feldman was successful enough that in July 1930 he figured in a plot that led to this top-line headline in *The Capital Times*: "$10,000 Extortion Plot Here Foiled." A disgruntled former employee mailed a letter demanding the money with the question, "What would a complete shut down mean to you?" Feldman turned the letter over to authorities and they made an arrest before the day was out.

Jacob Feldman's business success apparently did not carry over to his family life. An admiring 1930 front-page profile of Jacob in *The Capital Times* – published just a week before the extortion attempt – makes no mention of his wife, Molly, or daughters Elizabeth and Evelyn. Jacob and Molly eventually divorced, and their chilly relationship may have played a part in an episode that nearly brought a premature end to the courtship of

5. Elizabeth

Karl and Elizabeth, which began with the canoe ride date in July 1928.

Karl was a poetry-writing romantic, and he was smitten. Elizabeth was, too, but she was wary, having seen her mother's unhappiness in her marriage. Elizabeth also shared her mother's independent streak, which included Molly joining in 1923 the new Madison chapter of the Women's International League for Peace and Freedom. That group proclaimed for women "the right and responsibility to participate in decision-making on all aspects of peace and security."

In the fall of 1928, just a couple of months after Karl and Elizabeth's canoe ride, she took a trip to Europe. Elizabeth completed her undergraduate degree in the spring and the trip may have been a graduation present. She was an excellent student, having studied philosophy and been honored with induction into Phi Beta Kappa. By 1930 she received a second

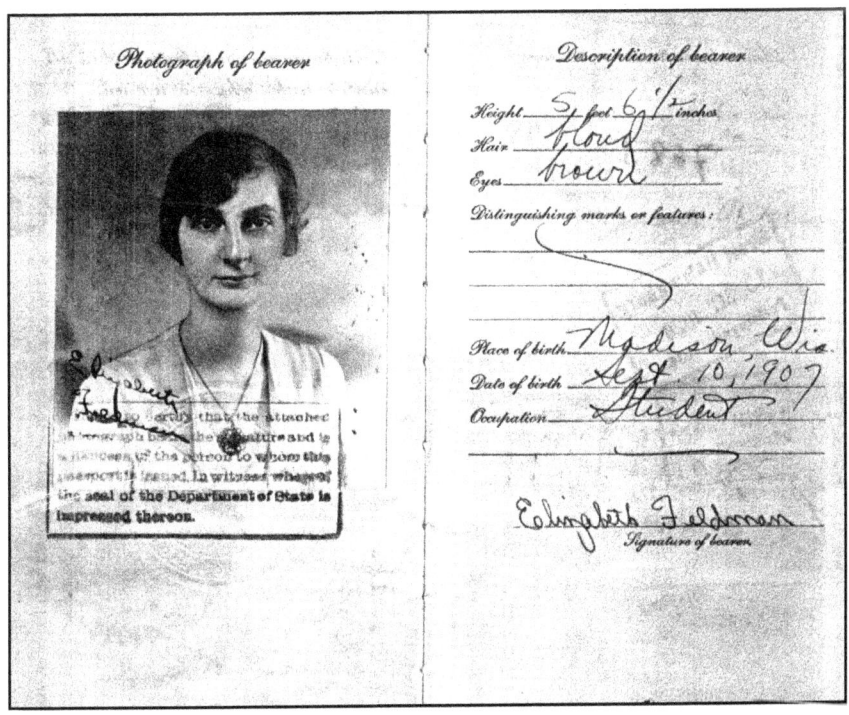

Elizabeth's passport photo. She traveled to Europe after graduating from the University of Wisconsin. (Link family).

degree from UW-Madison, a master's in German. On the eve of her leaving for Europe, Karl presented Elizabeth with a sheaf of papers – notes he'd written for her, to be read, one each day, on the Europe trip. It was charming and sentimental and maybe it was too much. Elizabeth enjoyed her time in Europe. She saw the Pope in Rome. She also acquired a German boyfriend.

Whatever the motivation, the relationship was not serious, yet when Karl learned of it – presumably in a letter – he was devastated.

"He carried that burden until the day he died," their son Tom said. "He just couldn't forgive her."

One can imagine Karl summoning the story years later, in moments of anger, but in fact he did get over it in the short term. They did not see each other immediately when Elizabeth returned to Madison, but a chance meeting led them, in son Tom's words, "to give it another try." They got back together, and despite ups and downs and those jagged shards of memory, they stayed together for the next 50 years. "I do know," Karl wrote Elizabeth in 1946, "that no woman was ever loved harder and more passionately than you by me."

Karl Paul Link and Elizabeth Feldman were married on Saturday, September 20, 1930 at Elizabeth's parents' home, 1601 Adams Street, not far from campus on Madison's west side. It was a small ceremony, without attendants, followed by an open house that evening.

While Karl and Elizabeth may have taken a brief honeymoon – their first residence was an apartment on Hawthorne Court, between State Street and University Avenue – they waited until December for a true getaway, a trip that took them to visit several members of Karl's family in Tucson, then to California and on up to Wyoming and Yellowstone National Park.

After Hawthorne Court, Karl and Elizabeth moved to a beautiful area on the western fringe of Madison called the Highlands. Their first Highlands home – built in 1931 – was a 16 by 24-foot cabin from which they could see both Lake Mendota

5. Elizabeth

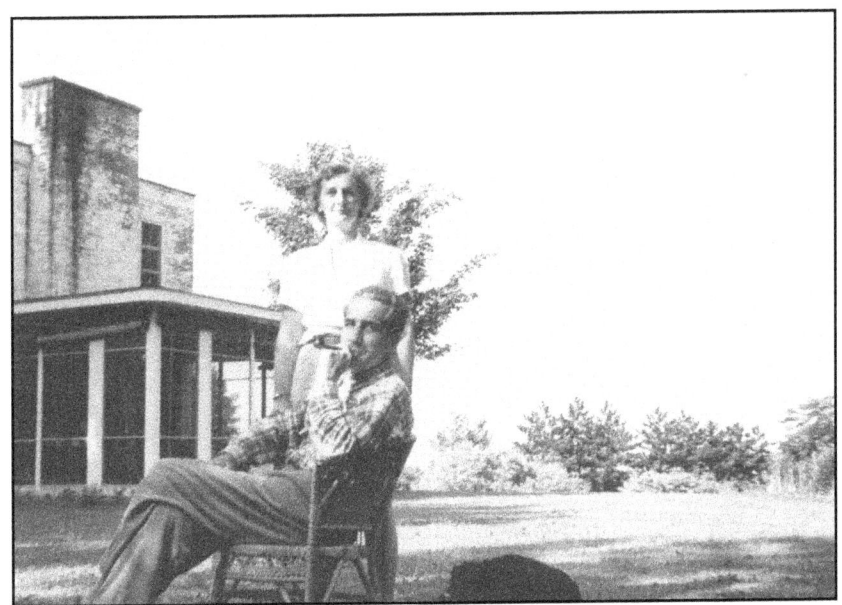

Karl and Elizabeth outside their home on Willow Lane, circa 1950. (Link family)

and the State Capitol Building. According to Don Behm, electricity was in place by 1932 and the couple lived in the cabin while their larger, permanent residence was being built. That home on Willow Lane – which would eventually be known as the Link Friendship House – was designed by Chicago architect Ernest Grunsfeld, whose works include the 1930 design for the Adler Planetarium in Chicago.

"The larger family home was built during 1933," Behm wrote, "and Elizabeth supervised the transplanting of flowering shrubs, trilliums, birches from the Wisconsin River, maples, and sycamores from La Porte, Indiana."

Burris added, "Karl grew legumes and plowed them under for a few years to build up soil before planting a lawn."

It appears Behm may have again been off by a year in terms of the home construction. Karl's archive includes a letter from J. W. Rose & Son of Madison offering an estimate of the cost of building the home. The letter is dated July 27, 1934.

"Dear Professor Link," it began, "I hereby submit to you an estimate of $8,140 for the erection of your house as per plans and specifications drawn by Ernest A. Grunsfeld, Jr."

The Highlands was then largely vacant land and woods, and in his unpublished memoir Karl noted that between 1931-34 he "used to do some 22 short rifle practice on Lot 11 Highlands." His companion was a UW radiologist who shot a 22 automatic. "I called him 'The Gay Dog' and he called me 'Horsie,'" Karl recalled, "for I was usually wisecracking or bullshitting while we practiced."

If Karl and Elizabeth by the early 1930s were hard at work establishing their new home in the Highlands, it was also a busy time for Karl on campus. After all, it was a day in February 1933 when farmer Ed Carlson came from northern Wisconsin to Madison with a dead cow and a bucket of blood, the visit that launched Karl on a yearslong quest to find what it was in the spoiled sweet clover that was causing Wisconsin dairy cows to hemorrhage.

But while Carlson's visit is rightly remembered as the trigger for Karl's work with anticoagulants – the work that made him famous – it should be noted he also spent time in the early 1930s working with hexuronic acids and carbohydrates.

"His publications in this area still serve as primary references in the field," noted Clint Ballou, a distinguished biochemist and former student of Karl's, in 1983.

"Link very nearly was the discoverer of vitamin C," said UW biochemist Dave Nelson, adding that there was essentially a "race" among scientists worldwide to identify the antiscorbutic agent that would cure scurvy.

"There were several people hot on the trail of the antiscorbutic agent," Nelson said. "I have set of notes of Link's all about the antiscorbutic factor. He had a lot of structural information. He was within months of being the one who discovered [vitamin C]. He wasn't just working on the sweet clover problem."

5. Elizabeth

Karl also hadn't abandoned carbohydrate chemistry work – certainly not in his teaching, whether in the undergraduate classroom or with graduates in the lab.

"It performed as an important vehicle for training graduate students," Ballou noted. (In 1943, when the UW's Department of Biochemistry sent a letter to Stockholm recommending Karl for the Nobel Prize in Chemistry, along with his anticoagulant breakthroughs they cited his work in "carbohydrate characterization – the identification of seven aldo-monosaccharides as benzimidazole derivatives.")

In Karl's archive there survives one of his Biochemistry 110 class exams on carbohydrates that would be meaningless to anyone but an advanced science student – except for the cover letter that Karl included with the exam. It offers a kind of shorthand guide to Karl's view of biochemistry and its teaching, and as such, is fascinating.

It begins with what Karl calls his "motto," a quote from the English mathematician Karl Pearson:

"The true aim of the teacher must be to impart an appreciation of method, an understanding of principles, and not a knowledge of facts."

Karl then wrote: "Biochemistry is something more than a compilation of empirical facts. Dictionaries, handbooks, and lexicons, not the memory, are the proper storehouses of isolated facts. The intellect is perfected not by knowledge but by exercise. The time needed for memorizing a vast medley of facts can be far more profitably spent in training the brain to think clearly and logically. It is more important to be able to relate a general formula or transformation back to first principles than to memorize a number of specific formulae without knowing from whence they come or what they mean.

"This examination," Karl concluded, "is not drafted to test your capacity to memorize – but on the contrary to ascertain your understanding of the basic principles of the carbohydrates and how to use these principles. Without the precise molecular architecture of organic chemistry biochemistry would have remained a 'schmier.'" It's signed, "K.P.L."

In the early 1930s, the Department of Agricultural Chemistry at the University of Wisconsin was one of the best, or perhaps the best, in the country. (The name change to Department of Biochemistry occurred in 1938, following a December 1937 vote by the faculty.) The early '30s line-up of scientists was akin to the 1927 Yankees' "Murderers' Row" batting order: Under chairman E. B. Hart were Stephen Babcock, Conrad Elvehjem, Harry Steenbock – large names in science and academia, or soon to be.

"They were probably at the time the most prominent department of biochemistry or agricultural chemistry in the country," Dave Nelson said. "There were a couple of other places, including Yale, that were looking for vitamins. So, it's not that there weren't others – but [Wisconsin] stood out as one of the top places in the country."

Karl held his own in that company. It likely didn't hurt that he was instrumental in bringing Paul Karrer – the Swiss scientist just a few years away from winning the Nobel Prize – to the Madison campus in September 1933. Karl, of course, had studied with Karrer during his time in Europe. Karrer spoke to the Wisconsin section of the American Chemical Society in Madison. Karl picked him up in Chicago and Karrer spent two nights at the Willow Lane home with Karl and Elizabeth. He also spent time with Karl's graduate students in the lab.

Over the years, the graduate students who signed on with Karl got their money's worth. Clint Ballou, who was one of them, noted: "Link supervised the studies of 43 master's students and of 55 who were awarded the doctorate in Biochemistry… It is a measure of the man that he left a standard in teaching, research and public service that will not soon be surpassed."

"You can find in Link's papers," Dave Nelson said, "information about all the students he took on. My impression is he took on quite a few students – mostly graduate students, not

5. ELIZABETH

post-docs, back then. He offered them a place in the laboratory and promised to help them. If you look at the notes of someone who had been in his lab, you see there was a daily consult between Link and the student to see how things were going. Link was very much a hands-on guy."

6. IN THE LAB

As the 1930s unfolded, no lab work was more important than anticoagulants and the search for the hemorrhagic agent. What had caused the cows to bleed to death? It marked a change for Karl, and according to Dave Nelson, it's not one he would have had to clear with the heads of the department.

"Not formally," Nelson said. "At that time, Hart was the head of the department and I'm sure he paid attention to this change. But, now as then, the chairman doesn't tell you what to study. It's up to you to find something that's fundable and important."

And as Nelson noted, "At that time, [Karl's] tools were just right for isolating natural products and identifying their structure. Link was the preeminent natural products chemist on the campus. If Ed Carlson [the farmer with the dead cow] had researched to find the perfect person, it would have probably been Link. Link had the farm background; he understood the economics of dairy farming in the north. People were losing their farms. So there was some incentive for Link to change direction."

Carlson's arrival in Madison in February 1933, and its impact on Karl, was introduced in the first chapter of this narrative. Karl's speech in New York City, in which he told the story, was quoted. It is far and away the best-known recitation of the story of Carlson and the cow's blood. It is reprinted in a book celebrating the 100th anniversary of the Biochemistry Department on campus. But in fact, on November 9, 1942, Karl gave a talk to the Madison Literary Club – he and Elizabeth had been members since 1932 – which offers even more personal detail on the circumstances of that day in February 1933.

6. In the Lab

The 1942 Literary Club speech was Karl's second to that group. He had addressed them in March 1934, in which he offered a brief history of the field of chemistry. In it, Karl quoted the German scientist Emil Fischer, whom Karl called "the most daring chemical virtuoso of all time."

Fischer, Karl said, stated: "The ultimate aim of biochemistry is to gain complete insight into the unending series of changes which attend plant and animal metabolism."

Eight years later, in 1942, Karl gave the club a vastly informative and entertaining talk about not only the Ed Carlson visit in February 1933, but how it sparked the search for an answer to the cow deaths and where that search finally led.

That Saturday noon, Karl said, he saw a man scanning the departmental directory of the Agricultural Chemistry Building. Karl immediately ascertained the man wasn't on a casual campus visit but rather serious business.

"He had a couple of milk cans beside him," Karl told the Literary Club. "I asked him if I could be of help. He indicated that he wanted the Vets Control Laboratory. I replied it was in Ag Hall up the court. Since my laboratory has few direct dealings with the farmers of this Great Commonwealth, I did not have specific basis for showing an interest in his mission. But I asked him what he had in the milk cans. He informed me that they contained blood from cattle that he had lost. He wanted to have the blood examined, since his vet had told him that the cattle had died from sweet clover disease, which he doubted. So he came to the university to let the professors decide."

Karl looked inside Carlson's cans.

"This isn't blood," Karl said. "This is water colored with red ink." If it was blood, why hadn't it congealed?

"No, Prof," Carlson said, pointing to a bucket, "this is the blood that I got from the inside of one of my cows." Pointing to the other bucket, he added, "This can contains blood that we tapped off from a blister on the shoulder of another."

Carlson then told Karl he had the sweet clover he'd been feeding his stock out in his truck, along with a dead cow.

Karl made some phone calls, including one to the departments of Veterinary Science and Animal Husbandry, looking for help for Carlson. It was a Saturday, the weather was terrible, and Karl reached only a janitor. By this time, as noted in the first chapter, Karl's assistant Schoeffel had arrived. They could do little but console Carlson, and around 4 p.m., he left, though he and Karl spoke on the phone the next morning.

On that call, Karl advised the farmer that his vet was probably right, he should quit feeding his cows the sweet clover hay.

"Is that all you can offer?" Carlson said. "I lost two more yesterday."

As Dave Nelson and others have noted, this episode had a profound effect on Karl.

"I became conscious of one cardinal fact," Karl told the Literary Club, "that we were faced with a challenge of the first order which affected a way of living, and which might eventually have some very far reaching repercussions in the field of blood chemistry."

The challenge became Karl's central professional focus. And it was a challenge.

Later, in his 1958 New York speech, Karl would say of the ensuing lab work, "Between that fateful Saturday in February 1933, and June 1939 [when Harold Campbell first isolated the hemorrhagic agent], a long and arduous trail was followed."

Karl noted (again in 1958) that their early examination of the spoiled sweet clover hay believed to cause the cow hemorrhaging involved "chemical extraction, separation, and isolation problems."

Karl continued, "This hay was indeed a kind of biochemical grab-bag and yielded many inactive products, some new, most of them old. But suffice it to state that many a seething and simmering hope did not become a reality. At times the hemorrhagic agent

6. IN THE LAB

appeared to hover before us like thistle down only to elude us like the will of the wisp."

More specifically, Karl noted: "Two fundamental issues confronted us. First, there was no chemical criteria available to establish the presence of the hemorrhagic agent. Therefore, a bioassay involving a small experimental animal (rabbits) offered the only practical means of appraising the anticoagulant activity of test hays and extracts prepared therefrom...

"The immediate prospects of developing a reliable bioassay were not bright;" Karl continued, "indeed, they were dark, 'dark like the inside of a cow.' We had not had previous experience with that complex problem – blood coagulation."

The difficult work proceeded slowly, and by early 1939, with the lab on the precipice of its breakthrough discovery, two early colleagues – W. L. Roberts and W. K. Smith – had moved on from the project. Karl's team of graduate students now included Harold "Campy" Campbell; Charles F. Huebner; Ralph Overman; and Mark A. Stahmann.

Campbell came from the University of Illinois and eventually went on to a long career with General Foods. Huebner was from Milwaukee and would go on to a distinguished career as a chemist with Ciba Pharmaceuticals (later Novartis); Overman was a University of Illinois graduate, and after leaving Madison joined the faculty at Cornell University and worked at New York Hospital (with eventual Link colleague Irving S. Wright), before an early death, age 37, in 1953. Stahmann was from Utah, and after graduating from Brigham Young University in 1936, was awarded a fellowship to the University of Wisconsin, where he became a prized student of Karl's.

Stahmann left Madison for a time in the 1940s but returned within a few years and became a lifelong member of the faculty. Stahmann's role in the anticoagulant story is important; his relationship with Link, complicated.

"He was Link's golden boy," Dave Nelson said. "Until it all went to hell."

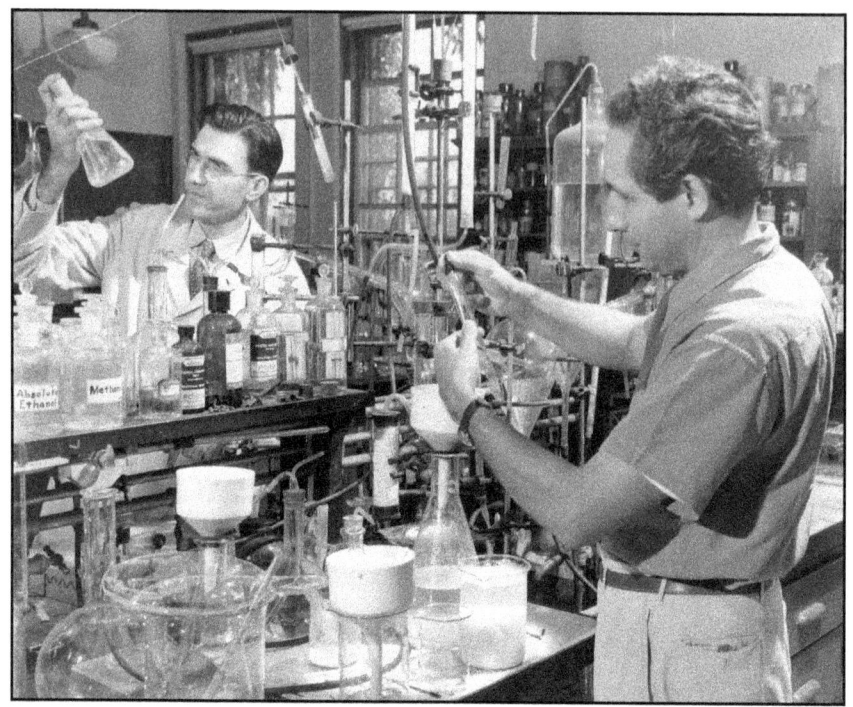

Karl, right, with Mark Stahmann, in a photo circa 1940.
The two would later have a serious falling out. (UW-Madison Archive)

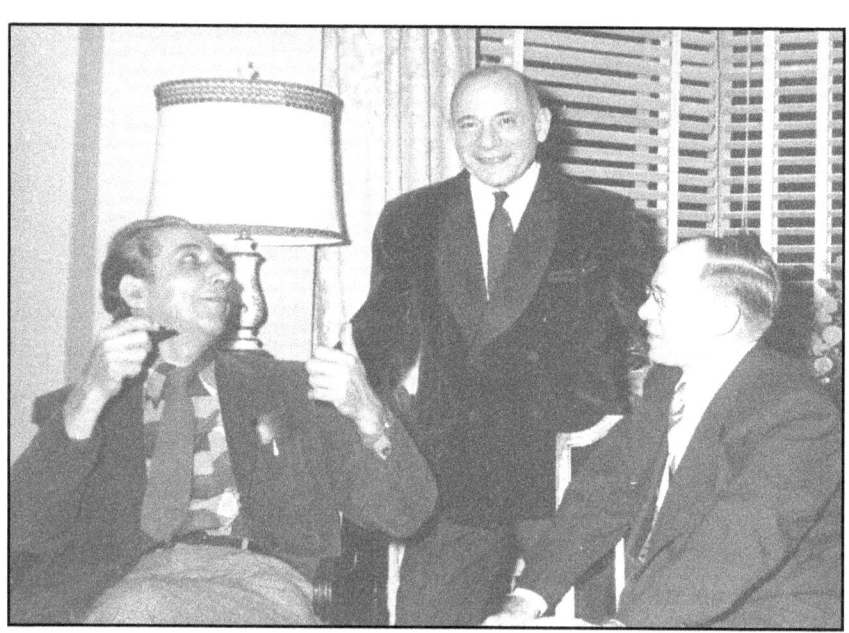

Karl, left, with colleagues Harold Campbell, right,
and Shepard Shapiro. (Link family)

6. IN THE LAB

That happened later, more than a decade after Stahmann's 1936 arrival in Madison. In the early years, Stahmann, like the rest of the graduate students, was excited to be in the Link lab. One reason, articulated later by a student in the department who was in a different lab, may have been the access to topflight equipment in Link's.

Henry Lardy – later a UW professor of biochemistry – told the University of Wisconsin Oral History Program: "[Link] had the best equipment in the department when I came as a student [circa 1939]. The work that was done on the isolation of dicumarol from sweet clover required a great deal of elaborate equipment and [Link] had it and knew how to use it."

Karl himself described his lab – and how he and his team worked – in some detail in his 1942 Literary Club talk.

"It is one of the best equipped and thoroughly appointed labs on the campus," Karl said, "having been sponsored originally by Deans Russell and Slichter via the Brittingham Funds. At the risk of being misinterpreted I am prepared to state that in this laboratory almost any chemical problem arising in agriculture can be attacked. I do not mean attacked with words or systems of abstract thinking, but experimentally.

"The number of workers is restricted to ten graduate students, all subsidized. They come from all over the country and diversification of talent is sought. Abraham Lincoln once said, 'It takes all kinds of animals to make up a good zoo.' Insofar as this lab might be likened to a zoo, we always have diverse and choice specimens. There is no formal class room teaching. Admittance is based on being able to demonstrate ability in the real as well as the abstract.

"The system of operation is communal," Karl said. "Lunch and tea come from the same table, there is a big cot (called the basket) for the necessary snoozes. The desks and quarters are kept trim by a series of divided assignments. To date the laboratory has never been graced by a female assistant. Hence it is sometimes stated, 'Link operates a monastery.' There is a discipline

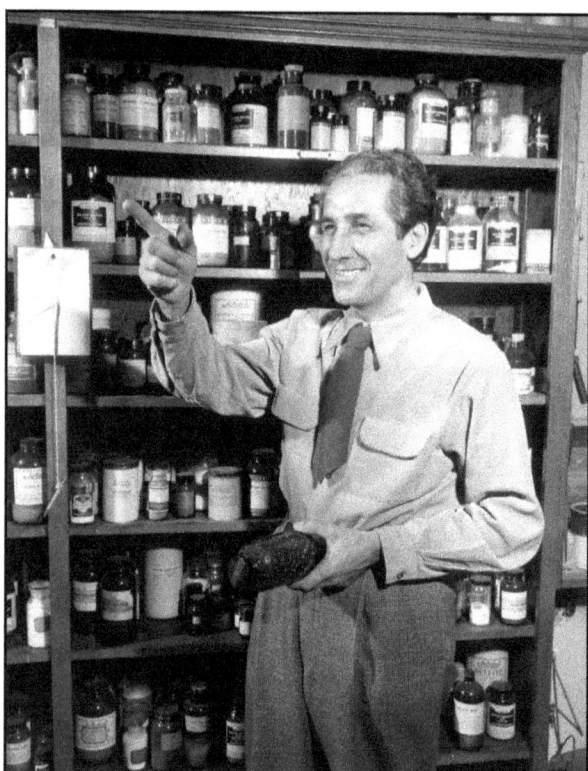

Karl in his lab. (UW-Madison Archive)

evident in this laboratory which the assistants maintain spontaneously.

"Most of them, by the way, are chosen from the B group. The hard road of experience has made us suspicious of the straight A students, since an undue amount of time is required to comb out the poetical fancies and the many uncorrelated useless facts that they carry in their brains. As Sherlock Holmes declared, 'It is a mistake to think that this little room (man's brain) has elastic walls and can distend to any extent. Depend on it.' Holmes warned, 'There comes a time when for every addition of new facts you forget something that you knew before. It is of the highest importance, therefore, not to have useless facts elbowing out the useful ones.'"

Karl concluded his description of his lab with this: "Problems are always attacked on a team basis. All conferences

6. IN THE LAB

work in open session, the whole crew might be assigned to the same problem if the circumstances warrant."

Karl provided a much lengthier, more detailed, and passionate window into his views on teaching and the laboratory six years earlier, in 1936, at a research discussion hour in the UW Biochemistry Lab. He was addressing his students directly. He called it his "horse-radish and vinegar speech."

Karl began: "There are at least four essentials for success in scientific work, and, as far as that goes, in any division of human activity. They are the following:

"1. You must have brains and you must be curious.
"2. You must have lots of steam.
"3. You must have some good breaks.
"4. You must know how to take the bad breaks."

Karl went on to tell the students they were accepted into his lab based on his appraisal of their record and in interviews and considering their letters of recommendation.

"I am by no means infallible and I have made mistakes in the appraisal of men who sought admission to this laboratory," Karl said. "I think I can state, without laying myself open to the accusation that I am boasting, that so far I have not denied admission to a good man when space permitted. To date all the mistakes have been on the other side – I erred by being too lenient – too much included to give the individual concerned the benefit of my doubts."

Some other highlights from the talk:

"You must have steam, drive if you wish (not mere potential ambition); and you must have lots of it. You must be right at the laboratory problem. It must not be at the periphery of your graduate student activities... I wish to emphasize a point that I hold to be very important and which is, in my opinion, being overlooked by some of you. A large factor in obtaining success is tied up with the fight or drive you put in at the very moment when failure begins to stalk in your path."

Karl invoked his work with Fritz Pregl:

"He was an artist driven by a demonic spirit that refused to accept defeat. He was also a great scientist. His methods represent more than mere refinements or scaling down of the classical macro methods. In many instances mere refining or scaling down led to defeat. New technique, new designs of apparatus, etc., were required. He had no breaks – in fact, the breaks were all against him. He had brains. He had steam – lots of it. He had a curiosity which refused to accept defeat.

"I want you fellows," Karl said, "to adopt the method of Pregl. If you can do so, I am sure that there is a place for you in this laboratory."

One might assume that teaching and the lab were Karl's life, but of course, they weren't, not entirely.

On October 5, 1934, Karl wrote a lengthy letter to Paul Karrer, the scientist who had mentored him in Zurich and then visited Madison in 1933. Karl began the letter to Karrer with an apology for not having written sooner, citing numerous factors, including a spring and summer drought in the Midwest that produced "terrific dust storms."

Karl noted, "The dust was so terrific that for two and a half days we could not see Lake Mendota from our place. The sun was scarcely visible and when it could be seen at high noon it appeared as a faintly yellow ball – as one would see the sun through a smoked glass."

The drought and dust eventually subsided, and what was truly keeping him busy, Karl wrote, was work on a new home on their Highlands property. Karrer had been a guest at the original – modest – cabin a year earlier.

"In August [1934]," Karl wrote, "Mrs. Link and I set out on the big task of building a new modern home. The work on the new home is progressing nicely now. It is located farther up near the crest of our hill – and has a gorgeous view of Lake Mendota.

6. IN THE LAB

We expect to get into the new house about January 1, 1935. We were fortunate in obtaining the services of a first-class architect of considerable fame in the United States, who developed the floor plan that I had worked out and who added the architectural unity that a home requires. He is Mr. Ernest Grunsfeld, the designer of the Adler Planetarium, which you will recall was readily visible on the lake front in Chicago. He was also the architect for several public buildings in Chicago (not skyscrapers) which are looked upon as first-class structures.

"Building a new house is quite an undertaking," Karl continued, "especially with the architect 150 miles away. This means that I have to do all the supervising of the construction and see to it that the plans and specifications are followed in detail. I really enjoy the work immensely but it does take a considerable amount of time. The task of becoming thoroughly familiar with all the plans and specifications is no small one in itself, let alone actually checking up on the various trades in the building process. The house itself is a brick tile masonry structure with brick as the outside."

Karl concluded, "You can well imagine that my hands have been more than full.... My early experiences while a student working in various factories and at different occupations had the decided advantage in that I became thoroughly familiar with the reading of plans and blueprints. Well, so much for that – when the house is finished I shall send you a picture of it."

The home construction was just one way that through the mid- to late 1930s, while Karl and his team were closing in on a discovery that would excite the medical world, life went on outside the lab.

In December 1936, Karl's sister-in-law, Elizabeth's sister, Evelyn, married Dr. Shepard Shapiro, in New York City. Elizabeth and her parents attended. Shapiro later worked with Karl on anticoagulants, especially studies of how vitamin K could counteract the effects of dicumarol and excessive bleeding. (Years later, after Shapiro's death in 1966, Karl wrote some notes of tribute, preserved in his archive, about Shapiro: "He took the oath of Hippocrates seriously. He was a healer. His patients adored him. He was also a seeker – he sought to prolong life.")

The following year, 1937, was for Karl one of both celebration and mourning. In May, his mother died in Tucson. She had outlived her husband by nearly a quarter century. A month later, on June 20, Karl and Elizabeth welcomed their first child, John Kailin, into the world. John was born at Wisconsin General Hospital, the precursor to the University of Wisconsin Hospital.

"Kailin," of course, was Elizabeth's mother's maiden name, and by the late 1930s, one of Elizabeth's first cousins, Clarence Kailin, was making newspaper headlines in Madison for his participation in the Spanish Civil War on the side of the anti-fascist Republican loyalists. Elizabeth, too, was passionately on the side of the Republicans, voicing her belief that the United States government should provide them economic aid.

Her cousin Clarence, meanwhile, joined the Abraham Lincoln Brigade to fight the fascists. A Madison resident, Clarence spent 22 months in Spain, returning to Madison in January 1939 having been seriously wounded by a machine gun bullet that severed an artery in his arm. He was outraged by the United States' professed neutrality, telling *The Capital Times* that by staying on the sideline "this nation must share the blame for helping Hitler and Mussolini win another victory for fascism."

Karl did what he could, too. A United Press story from December 1938, printed in the *Wisconsin State Journal*, began, "Some of America's foremost scientists raised their voices against 'the false and unscientific doctrine' of Nazism and Fascism..." The letter was signed by more than 1,200 scientists, including a number on the Madison campus. Among them: Karl Paul Link and Harry Steenbock.

Meanwhile, back in the lab, 1938 turned to 1939 without a solution to what in the sweet clover caused the cows to hemorrhage.

6. In the Lab

"At times it appeared to me," Karl told the Literary Club in 1942, "after five difficult years of labor, that my project leader, Campy [Harold Campbell], was standing on the brink of a vast obscurity, like a lonely figure on the shore of a turbulent gray ocean, which would never reveal the secret sought."

But Campbell, Karl continued, "was made of good stuff. Economic fortune had never smiled on this issue of the Campbell clan. But nature had been kind to him. He was one of those fortunate mortals who really knew nothing of indecision, much less of self-mistrust. In the darkest hours he could still say, 'Everything's OK. Things might be much worse.' Campbell has an alert and critical mind. He never hunted hares of his own raising. He had a special gift for deflecting interest from his personal speculative opinion to measurable fact.

"But Campy could grouse too," Karl continued. "He simply loathed attending most classes, and the remarks that he would make about some that he had to attend to attain the degree were very caustic. 'So-and-so is dead as mutton.'"

Campbell always kept a brush near his lab bench. On returning from a particularly dim lecture, he brushed off his shoes, saying he was getting rid of the academic dust.

"But he groused only for a moment," Karl said. "The next he was at the bench, working."

It was 2:30 a.m. on June 28, 1939, Karl said, when Campy saw something in a test tube and put it under the microscope. It was the holy grail, the hemorrhagic agent. As noted in the first chapter, Campbell waited a day or so to tell Karl. In his 1942 Literary Club address, Karl recalled the big moment a bit differently than he did subsequently in New York in 1958.

He told the Literary Club that Campbell came to see him and said, "How long can you afford to run this project at the rate we're going?"

Karl (who knew what Campy was about to tell him), said flippantly, "One hundred years."

"Well," Campbell said, "you won't have to wait that long. Here she is, crystalline, named H. A. for hemorrhagic agent."

It was fitting that a favorite test rabbit, Walt – named for the poet Walt Whitman – had provided the assay that produced the breakthrough.

Campbell soon had to leave the lab for a full-time job, while the challenge of synthetically reproducing the natural product in the lab remained. Its chemistry needed to be determined. It would have been customary to turn the material over to organic chemists, the experts at molecular structure. Karl was not inclined to turn over the hard-won hemorrhagic agent to anyone; besides, he had organic chemistry expertise in his lab in the persons of Charlie Huebner and Mark Stahmann.

Karl explained his thinking to the Literary Club in 1942: "Turn H. A. over to another lab? Not on your life!" Karl said. He described Huebner and Stahmann. "Huebner is a minute of a man in stature, but quick-witted. Using Professor McElvain's phrase, 'He's as good as they come' and is always referred to by the boys as 'the mighty Charlie.' Stahmann in contrast is a big Mormon barge from Spanish Fork, Utah, a veritable horse for work."

They were charged with making Campbell's isolated discovery synthetically. Likely the best and most concise description of what followed is contained in a letter written by Karl to Chris Christensen, dean of the College of Agriculture, summarizing their efforts in 1939-40.

Karl wrote: "I am sure that you will be glad to learn that the combined efforts of Messrs. Harold Campbell, Ralph Overman, Charles Huebner, and Mark Stahmann have led to the elucidation of the chemical structure of the hemorrhagic agent present in spoiled sweet clover hay, and to its synthesis from known starting products."

Karl then tells Christensen about Campbell's June 1939 isolation of the hemorrhagic agent, adding that when Campbell left the lab that October, Charlie Huebner and Mark Stahmann

6. In the Lab

took over. Karl notes that in April 1940, they delivered an artificial, or synthesized, version of the hemorrhagic agent.

"The chemical and physical properties," Karl wrote, "were in full agreement with the naturally occurring product."

In the Christensen letter, Karl left out the colorful details of how he learned of Huebner and Stahmann's success. He shared the story in his 1942 Literary Club talk.

Karl was in club car cabin – this was early April 1940 – headed for a speaking engagement in Ames, Iowa. The train was the *City of Denver*. It was 9:30 at night, Karl was chatting with some Colorado cattlemen about sweet clover hay. During a stop at Clinton, Iowa, a voice barked: "Telegram for Professor Link!"

Karl reached for it, saying, "And now what has my son John done? Just last week, he ate some glass."

One of the cattlemen said, "What did you do, Doc?"

"Mrs. Link called the doctor and I suggested he be given a lot of bread. He survived."

The telegram – signed "Charlie and Mark" – brought the news of their success synthesizing the hemorrhagic agent.

Karl set the message down in the club car and announced he was buying a round. "Porter, set up this house!"

In his letter to Dean Christensen, Karl noted: "The crew," as Karl called his lab assistants, "is also engaged at present with the preparation of synthetic analogues with higher prothrombin [clot]-destroying powers… It appears that one of the compounds made to date exerts its prothrombin-destroying powers more rapidly than the aforementioned substance. Arrangements will be made to survey the application of our hemorrhage inducing substances to medical practice."

As noted in the first chapter, the first public mention, some months later in November 1940, of the breakthrough, in a University of Wisconsin news release that was picked up with little fanfare by *The Capital Times*, did note its possible import for humans:

"Because it is very potent in preventing the coagulation of blood, it may have value in treating diseases caused or complicated by blood clots."

Karl ended his letter to Dean Christensen with this:

"In closing it gives me great pleasure to state that all of the chemical and biochemical work done on this problem during the past five years has been executed by regular station assistants in the process of training for the Ph.D. degree."

Four months after the short, low-key "Solve Mystery of Disease in Cattle" story in *The Capital Times*, Karl and his team and their laboratory success hit the big time – for Madison, anyway – with a lengthy, front-page, Sunday edition *Wisconsin State Journal* story, March 9, 1941, headlined: "UW Research on Clover Brings Blood Discovery." The secondary headline read: "May Have Medical Importance Around the World."

There was a large photograph of Karl, and another of, as the photo caption read, "the four 'team' members who have helped 'Coach' Karl Paul Link in the years of research leading to chemical analysis of di-coumarin compound." The four were Mark Stahmann, Charlie Huebner, Ralph Overman and a newcomer, William Sullivan, who would earn his doctorate in 1942.

The article took a cautionary tone toward the potential medical benefits for humans – "the time for its general use in medicine is a long way off," said a UW Medical School doctor – but in fact, clinical trials began just weeks after the article appeared, at UW-Madison, the Mayo Clinic, and New York University, the latter under the auspices of Dr. Shepard Shapiro.

Karl understood that physicians would determine the discovery's medical future. In his 1942 remarks to the Literary Club, he said, "Biochemists should be bold in experiment – but cautious in their claims."

It was up to the medical people. Before long – by August 1941 – doctors at the Mayo Clinic were ready to announce some very exciting news.

7. DICUMAROL

THE FIRST NEWS OF 1941 was personal – the birth, in January, of a second son to Karl and Elizabeth.

Among those sending congratulatory notes about the boy, whom they named Thomas, was Max Bergmann, a member of the Rockefeller Institute for Medical Research in New York City, and its top protein scientist. Bergmann was born in Bavaria and was a distinguished scientist in Germany until 1934, when, with the rise of Adolph Hitler, he left that country for the United States. Bergmann and Karl shared both professional respect and a warm friendship, one that was furthered in 1939 when Karl encouraged Bergmann to bring one of Karl's students, Stanford Moore, to the Rockefeller Institute. Bergmann did invite Moore, who accepted and remained there throughout his distinguished career, which included a Nobel Prize in 1972.

"Heartiest congratulations to Elizabeth, John and yourself on your unfinished protein symphony," Bergmann wrote in a Western Union telegram to Karl in January 1941. "I hope mother [and baby] are well."

Baby Tom had been born early in Florida while Elizabeth was visiting her father, Jacob Feldman, who owned a home in Hollywood, between Miami and Fort Lauderdale. Her visit was extended after young Tom spent his first few weeks in the hospital. In April, Elizabeth sent Karl a letter in Madison saying they'd be returning shortly. (Karl had been in Florida with Elizabeth and John prior to Tom's unexpected arrival, but needed to return to his lab in Madison.)

Elizabeth's letter was affectionate, filled with tidbits about their newborn and written, at least in part, in response to a letter Karl sent after attending a conference in Chicago. He mentioned having met a biochemistry professor from the University of Toronto named Hermann Otto Laurenz Fischer, son of Emil Fischer, the German Nobel Prize-winning organic chemist in whose lab in Germany Max Bergmann had worked.

"Dearest Karl," Elizabeth began her response. "Thank you for your delightful letter of Friday. It came this noon to my intense joy."

Of meeting Fischer, Elizabeth wrote, "There must be a hallowed feeling when one first meets him knowing him to be the blood of the great Emil… Was Max Bergmann there?"

The balance of Elizabeth's letter was about the baby, apparently nicknamed "Pelican."

"I have decided to see if we can't work out a [unintelligible word] feeding schedule for Pelican which will eliminate all night feedings. This should be easy to manage because he's such a plump little cherub… He is developing every minute. Just a few moments ago when I went in to change his pants, he laughed out loud when I touched his tummy – and his face dimpled."

Elizabeth closed with this: "Goodbye Darling. We'll be with you soon… We love you so much. Your own Lisa."

Much was happening, and quickly, in Karl's professional life as well. He said later it took him by surprise how swiftly medical clinicians began their investigation of the anticoagulant compound that eventually became known as dicumarol.

In a February 1941 speech to the Wisconsin Medical Society, Karl had acknowledged that while they were excited about the prospects for their lab discovery, the clinicians would render the final judgment.

"We are now at the beginning of things [with the anticoagulant compound]," Karl said, "and not at the end, as chemists are prone to conclude after the molecular structure of a compound is solved."

7. DICUMAROL

The *Wisconsin State Journal* story that essentially introduced the work of Karl and his team to the world ran a month later, in March 1941. According to Don Behm's biographical essay on Karl, the compound had been turned over to the clinicians a few months earlier – "in late 1940." By summer 1941, Mayo Clinic went public with some trial results.

An August 2, 1941 Associated Press story, datelined Rochester, had this opening: "Medical use of a new chemical discovered in sweet clover, which delays clotting of human blood, has been announced in the proceedings of the Mayo Clinic.

"The clover remedy shows promise," the story continued, "for treating a variety of difficult diseases, including thrombosis, the blood clots which lodge in heart or lungs and often cause death... They tried it on dogs and found something remarkable, namely, no bad effects of any kind. They then used it on six human patients, with equally remarkable absence of untoward effects. The only other similar remedy, the recently discovered heparin, a liver extract, sometimes has made patients ill."

Two decades later, in a national radio interview for the program "Men and Molecules," produced by the American Chemical Society, Karl addressed the initial clinical trials.

"To our surprise, and somewhat to our consternation," Karl said, "it was taken up quite rapidly by clinicians for the purpose of fighting complications and diseases that involved blood clots in the human system.

"Did we think of that when we started the project?" Karl said. "The answer to that is no. I can say, however, that beginning about 1938, '39, after we were on the project five or six years, it dawned upon us that this substance that killed cattle might find a use to prevent clots in human medicine. It must be said to the everlasting credit of the medical profession, it took us very little time lost between our fundamental work and what we thought we could do and their checking it clinically to see whether or not the compound would behave in man as it did through overdosage in cows."

Karl concluded, "The two men who were largely responsible for promoting what you might call anti-coagulant therapy in the United States were Dr. Edgar Allen of the Mayo Clinic, and Dr. Irving Wright of the Cornell Medical College."

Initially, in a fascinating correspondence with Karl in August 1941, Wright was somewhat skeptical (though always hopeful) of the benefits of dicumarol use in humans. The tone of their letters back and forth is also noteworthy. It is highly respectful.

Wright was then a physician and executive officer in the Department of Medicine at the New York Post-Graduate Medical School of Columbia University. Wright himself – in 1938 – had been "gravely ill" (according to a later *New York Times* story) with thrombophlebitis, which causes blood to clot and block veins. He had a heightened interest in anticoagulants and had already worked with heparin when Karl sent him a paper his team had produced titled "Studies on Hemorrhagic Sweet Clover Disease," which told the dicumarol story. Wright, as it turned out, had already been working with the compound. He began his letter by thanking Karl for sending the dicumarol paper.

"It is a very comprehensive and significant paper," Wright wrote Karl in a letter dated, August 13, 1941. "We have been using the material on about 15 patients, and although we have given relatively small doses as compared with the Mayo Clinic report, we have had some rather severe hemorrhages, details of which I will forward to you in the near future."

Wright continued: "It has also convinced me that the preparation should not be released to the general medical public, or even to large groups of workers at this time. I feel that this is a potentially valuable substance, but it may fall into disrepute if a few deaths occur as a direct result of its use...

"I have already heard of some men in general practice, who without adequate laboratory facilities, are attempting to use it clinically. It appears to me that this is a very risky procedure at

7. DICUMAROL

the present time, and I am anxious to hear whether you are in accord with my views on this subject.

"I wish to keep in very close touch with you," Wright concluded. "Your animal studies are an invaluable help in guiding us as to methods of approach in man."

Karl replied to Wright's letter immediately. In a letter dated August 16, 1941, Karl thanked Wright, saying he was "particularly grateful for your cautious approach to the problem at hand." Karl then quoted from his February speech to the Wisconsin Medical Society saying they were at "the beginning" of the process.

Karl and Wright were on the cusp of a beneficial collaboration as well as a warm friendship.

Wright wrote back quickly. "It is a great pleasure to work with a man in one of the more functional fields, who has such a full appreciation of the clinical problems involved in the type of research which we are attempting to pursue."

Wright was also friendly with Edgar Allen, the physician leading the dicumarol study at Mayo. In an August 20 letter to Karl, Wright quoted a letter sent to him by Allen: "We have seen no harm at all in the use of coumarin compound, but I don't doubt that there will be some trouble sometime."

Allen added, in his letter to Wright, "I am thoroughly in accord with the feeling expressed in your letter to Dr. Link."

So in late summer 1941, the medical and scientific communities' attitude toward dicumarol use in humans was one of cautious optimism. It is worth remembering, in reading this early correspondence, that 19 years later, in 1960, these three men – Karl, Wright, and Allen – would share the prestigious Lasker Award for their work with oral anticoagulants. (Karl had individually received a Lasker Award in 1955 for his pioneering research in anticoagulants.)

That fall – on October 11, 1941 – an application was filed with the United States Patent Office on behalf of Karl Paul Link, Mark Stahmann, Harold Campbell, and Charles Huebner for the compound known as dicumarol, "an anticoagulant which is suitable for administration to man."

While that application was eventually withdrawn and reworked into a different application, it did establish what is called priority of invention.

Equally important to note is who filed the patent: the Wisconsin Alumni Research Foundation (WARF), on behalf of the four scientists.

Karl would have a long, at times rewarding, and at times exasperating, relationship with WARF, which was established in 1925, largely through the efforts of Harry Steenbock, a UW scientific colleague of Karl's and, with time, an unfriendly rival.

In the early 1920s, Steenbock, working with rats in his laboratory, found that if he generated the symptoms of rickets – a crippling bone disease caused by a deficiency of vitamin D, especially debilitating to children – he could rid the rats of the disease by providing them food that had been treated with artificial ultraviolet light. The breakthrough, once perfected and applied to people, led noted science writer Paul de Kruif to say Steenbock, in helping cure rickets, had "trapped the sun."

According to an unpublished history of WARF written by UW journalism professor Clay Schoenfeld, Steenbock was reluctant to simply commercialize his discovery because of the earlier experience on the UW-Madison campus of Professor Stephen Babcock.

"Several decades earlier," Schoenfeld wrote, "Babcock had invented a revolutionary new test for the butterfat content of milk that ultimately would win worldwide acceptance. He chose not to patent the process but to 'give it freely to the world.' However, Babcock discovered that without patent rights he had no way to control the standards of accuracy or reliability of the test that carried his name. Moreover, there were financial benefits from its use which did not accrue to the inventor, the University, or the people of Wisconsin."

7. DICUMAROL

But according to WARF historian Dr. Kevin Walters (who did his doctoral dissertation on Steenbock), Steenbock's main motivation in seeking a patent on his vitamin D discovery (which led to the founding of WARF) was a larger desire to protect the Wisconsin dairy industry, the goodwill and political support of which had benefited science at the UW. Steenbock did not want his plant-based discoveries to yield a better margarine.

"Steenbock filed for patents to protect the dairy industry from fortified margarine," Walters noted. "He was then accused of betraying Babcock's generous example [of not patenting his buttermilk fat content test]. Steenbock responded to his critics that Babcock had been mistaken not to patent."

Steenbock, on the advice of a Chicago attorney, filed a U.S. patent application June 30, 1924. He paid $300 of his own money, when the UW Regents turned him down, according to Schoenfeld, "after the State Attorney General had ventured an informal opinion that the Regents were probably not so empowered to spend public monies."

Around the same time, after published reports suggested an association between eating oatmeal and developing rickets, Quaker Oats offered to buy the rights to the process – by some accounts, offering $1 million. Steenbock declined. Instead, he met with campus colleagues, administrators and attorneys. They considered various options, until Carl Miner, a chemist who had done consulting work for Quaker, showed Steenbock a published article outlining a nonprofit, patent-management corporation operated by "friends of the university."

After much handwringing, debate and pontificating, on and off the UW-Madison campus, WARF was established in 1925, using the "friends" proposal as a model and prominent UW alumni as the founding trustees.

Originally, WARF worked with individual inventors to patent and license their inventions, and in 1968, WARF became the designated patenting and licensing organization for UW-Madison. Its mission: To support, encourage and aid scientific research at the university. It was perhaps the first of what are now called technology transfer units that exist on, or (as is the case with WARF), in association with university campuses across the country. At UW, the money earned from commercializing the campus innovations is split among the scientists (who get a smaller percentage), and WARF, which over the decades has built a staggering investment portfolio worth $3 billion and annually provides UW-Madison with tens of millions of dollars in grants. (According to Walters, WARF ultimately signed a contract with Quaker Oats for $990,000. Whether $1 million was ever offered Steenbock – prior to the establishment of WARF – has not been documented.)

Karl worked closely with WARF on the patenting and licensing of both dicumarol, and, later, warfarin (named for WARF and coumarin), a stronger derivative that would be used to great financial success as both a rat poison and human anticoagulant.

Karl's archive includes voluminous papers related to his dealings with WARF, which, as noted, were a mixed bag. The scientist and the foundation were undeniably good for one another. Still, there was tension. Karl was a natural anti-authoritarian, and along with its many benevolent functions, WARF represented authority. As Dave Nelson said in his campus lecture on the 75th anniversary of warfarin's discovery, "Link had a tendency to antagonize the people around him." Nelson then showed a brief eight-millimeter film clip – unearthed by Karl's son, Tom – showing Karl grinning and throwing corn cobs at a building. It's the WARF headquarters.

In Karl's archive there is a folder with papers detailing the royalties he received from WARF through its patenting of dicumarol. The years covered are 1944-1961. Among the commercial licensees were Abbott Laboratories and Eli Lilly.

The net royalties are listed as $137,041.44. (It's important to remember that these are mid-20th-century dollars; and that the royalties for warfarin were considerably more substantial.)

7. Dicumarol

WARF also listed "development expenses prior to 1944" of more than $18,000, which were subtracted from the royalties. Karl received 15 percent of that adjusted figure, or a little over $22,000. The same folder contains a "statement of consulting fees" paid to Karl by WARF for the years 1951-1962. The total amount: $36,000. That amount, however, was adjusted by two line-item expenses attributed to Karl: $44.88 for a ladder, and $156.96 for a Smith Corona electric portable typewriter.

On the typed statement saved in his archive, Karl made a handwritten asterisk next to the ladder and typewriter expense lines. An asterisk at the bottom of the page then offers his handwritten assessment of the charges: "The cheap $$ grubbers."

As noted, the first dicumarol patent was filed in fall 1941. A few months later, in January 1942, Karl heard from his friend Max Bergmann at the Rockefeller Institute in New York City. Bergmann was looking for an assistant and had inquired about Mark Stahmann, who arrived in Madison in 1936 and was by early 1942 doing postdoctoral work in Karl's lab. Stahmann, of course, was one of the four names on the first patent application in 1941.

Karl's generous reply to Bergmann's inquiry about Stahmann is notable in part because before the decade of the 1940s was out, Karl and Stahmann would have a serious falling out.

Of Stahmann, Karl wrote in 1942, "There is no denying the fact that Stahmann is not as brilliant in his thinking as [Carl] Niemann [another of Karl's graduate assistants], nor as logical and systematic as Stan [Moore, Karl's student who would later win the Nobel Prize]. But the simple facts of the case are that the Big Mormon [Stahmann] has rung up a performance here that makes him score high. I sometimes wonder if Niemann and Stan working jointly would have elucidated the structure of the spoiled hemorrhagic agent any quicker than Mark and Charlie [Huebner] did.

"In short, I feel that he is a very good risk for you; that he is still in the upswing period, and that he would leave no stone unturned to meet the trust involved, from your side and mine."

Bergmann invited Stahmann to join him at the Rockefeller Institute, where Stahmann spent a little under three years, including conducting research for the U.S. military on toxic mustard gases.

In early 1942, around the time he was helping Stahmann secure the position with Bergmann, Karl was invited to give an address on his anticoagulant research at the Mayo Clinic in Rochester. The *Wisconsin State Journal* in Madison took note with an editorial that pointed out how rare it was for a non-medical professional to be asked to speak at Mayo.

"When a man is so good that others in his field listen to his counsel, that's grand," the *State Journal* opined. "When a man is so good that others outside his field ask for his counsel, that's both grand and amazing."

Karl's wife, Elizabeth, meanwhile, agreed in April 1942 to serve on the executive committee (as executive secretary) of the Madison chapter of Russian War Relief, Inc., which raised funds for medical supplies for Russian civilians impacted by the war in Europe. It was the early stages of Elizabeth's lifelong devotion to better U.S.-Russia relations, in service of an even larger goal of a peaceful world.

In October 1943, Elizabeth led an effort by the Madison chapter to find 50 women who would donate one afternoon a week for four weeks to repair clothing donated by people in Madison for Russian war relief. In an interview, Elizabeth told the *Wisconsin State Journal* that one-third of the goal of 30,000 pounds of clothing needed repair, and quickly, if the clothing was to be shipped before winter. (Not everyone appreciated Elizabeth's efforts. By 1946, she was acting secretary of a new group, the Madison Council of American-Soviet Friendship. The national organization came under fire from the House Un-American Activities Committee, or HUAC. Elizabeth responded

7. DICUMAROL

in a lengthy letter to the *State Journal* that the paper published under the headline, "Who's Un-American?" Elizabeth called HUAC's stance "a threat to civil liberties and to our friendly relations with the Soviet Union.")

In January 1944, Karl gave one of his most famous addresses – Behm, in his biographical essay on Karl, called it "celebrated."

It was a story he had told before – the title of the address was "The Anticoagulant from Spoiled Sweet Clover Hay" – but the setting made it special. It was Caspary Auditorium at Rockefeller University in New York City, at the invitation of the Harvey Society. The "Harvey Lectures" – the society was founded in 1905 – rank as one of the most distinguished lecture series worldwide.

Harvey speakers were expected to wear tuxedoes, indeed it was "mandatory," as one of Karl's students, Saul Roseman, later recalled. Instead, Karl "compromised by wearing a red vest with brass buttons under the jacket," Roseman said.

Karl began his address with a respectful thank you and just a bit of his usual sporting irreverence:

"I should like to express to the Harvey Committee my personal thanks and that of my students for inviting me here. My pleasure and surprise must also be indicated at finding so many interested in spoiled sweet clover. I had no idea that Manhattan and its environs harbored that many country gentlemen.

"Since I am a man of the soil," Karl continued, "trained as an agriculturist, I shall not aspire to that sustained intellectual effort exemplified by the Harvey lectures of my distinguished predecessors. In a sense I shall break with tradition tonight, and not lecture to you. Instead I shall tell you a story."

The dicumarol story, familiar now to readers of this narrative, had by early 1944 an additional component: Link's exasperation at the failure of at least some clinicians to accept his lab's finding that vitamin K – for the Danish word Koagulation, which is essential for blood clotting in animals – could counteract the effects of dicumarol. It was an important aspect of treatment for patients who might experience excessive bleeding after taking the anticoagulant. Vitamin K, Karl and his team believed, solved the problem.

In his 1958 address at the New York Academy of Medicine, Karl recalled his irritation at the initial confusion.

"When we turned dicumarol over to clinicians in the years 1940 to 1942," Karl said, "one significant point, clearly established by our work, was at first missed, in fact denied. I have reference to the capital fact that vitamin K (all forms – some better than others) can counteract the action of dicumarol.

"I emphasized this in letters, personal conversations, and in my first lectures on dicumarol at the Mayo Clinic and at Wisconsin General Hospital," Karl continued. "In spite of these efforts the first clinical reports carried the statement that 'vitamin K has no effect as an antidote to the administration of dicumarol.' The editorial and annotation writers for the medical journals, those who only 'think' but don't 'try,' innocently reiterated this statement.

"While in error, the clinicians were in good company, for an authority of blood coagulation [A.J. Quick] had written in 1937, and again in his book published in 1942, that 'vitamin K will not restore the prothrombin [necessary for clotting] concentration' depleted by dicumarol."

Karl said that while this circumstance made him "very unhappy" – he was in effect being accused of error – his greater concern was that a stigma would be attached to dicumarol that it was dangerous. "This did happen," Karl noted.

In his 1958 lecture, Karl said he was sustained by his belief that in science, "the truth will conquer." And indeed, scientists – notably Dr. Shepard Shapiro in New York City – began clinical trials that sustained Karl's claims for vitamin K as an antidote to the anticoagulant action of dicumarol. It is doubtless one reason why Karl spoke admiringly of Shapiro over the years.

7. Dicumarol

Around the time of Karl's 1944 Harvey lecture, the *Drug Trade News* published an article that announced dicumarol was "being manufactured and sold under license from the Wisconsin Alumni Research Foundation by four companies in the United States and two in Canada," and also noted "if required, the action of dicumarol can be suppressed with great ease. Dr. Shepard Shapiro and coworkers first showed in man that synthetic vitamin K, at high dosage levels, will counteract dicumarol."

In his biographical essay on Karl, Don Behm noted, "Later, a more reliable standard for assessing a patient's response to [dicumarol] and adjusting the dosage of oral anticoagulants was introduced with Dr. Shapiro's assistance and became known as the 'Link-Shapiro Method.'"

In the Harvey lecture, Karl noted that his lab did not stop after it successfully synthesized dicumarol – hardly. Inside of two years, more than 100 related coumarins were synthesized, without biochemical appraisal. They were grouped based on their chemical structure and assigned numbers. Who knew what they might portend?

Within a few years, one of those coumarins – number 42 – would be famous. It took a lengthy stay in a sanitarium for Karl before that happened. It resulted in the disintegration of Karl's relationship with a former student and once-valued colleague, Mark Stahmann. Perhaps the tumult should not be surprising, for coumarin number 42 rocked the world. Karl gave it its name – warfarin.

8. THE ROAD TO WARFARIN

ON NOVEMBER 7, 1944, Max Bergmann, age 58, good friend to Karl Paul Link and employer at the Rockefeller Institute of Mark Stahmann, died in Mount Sinai Hospital in New York City.

Almost immediately, Karl sent a letter to Stahmann, offering his assistance should Stahmann be looking to relocate. The institute's general practice was to disband divisions when the head man died or retired.

On November 22, Stahmann wrote back, thanking Karl "for your kind offer."

Stahmann noted that if he were to leave the institute, his preference was for a "university or Agricultural Experiment Station post," and that he was "still interested in plant chemistry."

In a return letter – sent December 1 – Karl wrote, "Perhaps I need not emphasize the fact that satisfactory positions in this category are amongst the rarest posts. However, I will be happy to do whatever I can to see this ambition realized."

Karl tempered this cautionary observation with a kind offer: "First of all I should perhaps indicate that you should not worry about the prospects of actually being out of a job. I have had an authorization for a $5,000 grant from the Corn Industries Research Foundation (for work on starch) in my files for over 2 years which can be put into operation any time I am ready to do so."

Calling Stahmann "my friend," Karl then notes that he also has correspondence from the Sugar Research Foundation about them potentially sponsoring a post-doctorate fellowship for work on beet pectin.

8. The Road to Warfarin

"I am glad," Karl wrote Stahmann, "that I have this kind of insurance on file for you."

Karl went further. The same day – December 1 – that he answered Stahmann's letter, Karl wrote to a friend of his who was an executive with General Foods Corporation, recommending Stahmann for a job. "I can underwrite Mark without reservations," Karl wrote.

In his December 1 letter to Stahmann, Karl concluded by suggesting Stahmann give serious thought to returning to UW-Madison.

Stahmann answered on December 11. "It is needless for me to say," he wrote near the end of a lengthy letter in which he discussed various options, "that Trudy [his wife] and I know of no place we'd enjoy making our home more than in Madison. If something attractive to me and satisfactory to both the Biochemistry and Plant Pathology Departments can be worked out, I would be very pleased."

It didn't happen immediately – Stahmann went to the Massachusetts Institute of Technology, where he helped establish a lab to develop antimalarial drugs – but eventually it did.

Stahmann's return to Madison coincided with a recurrence of Karl's tuberculosis. In his 1958 New York Academy of Medicine address, Karl explained how it happened:

"Early in September 1945, I was fed up with laboratory work, etc., and I went off on a canoe trip with my family. On this trip we were caught in a cold rainstorm. I got soaked and overexhausted. Two weeks later I came down with what I had had once before – after a similar heavy physical bout, as a student in Switzerland – wet pleurisy. At first my doctor thought I had pneumonia; then I told him about my previous bouts of tuberculosis; so the diagnosis was changed to reactivated pulmonary tuberculosis."

Karl was admitted to Wisconsin General Hospital, and then after a period of about two months, was transferred to the Lake View Sanitorium.

Karl later wrote: "What a moment – November 27, 1945 – to leave kith and kin to enter a sanitorium tipped with the double cross of Lorraine!"

As he so often did throughout his life, Karl stirred things up at Lake View. The sanitorium, opened in 1930, sat high on a hill in the town of Westport, outside Madison. With 105 beds, Lake View was considered state of the art for tubercular patients when it opened.

Admitted 15 years later, Karl was not impressed. His chief complaint seems to have been Lake View's practice of isolating tubercular patients, a practice, he noted, that countries in other parts of the world had begun to change.

Karl's review of his Lake View experience – he went home April 19, 1946 – was published in *Lake Views*, an in-house publication apparently written and edited by patients – certainly not the sanitorium administration. It billed itself as "a patient's free press."

Karl's piece was the lead article in the April 1946 issue. He called it "As Seen from 214" – his room number at Lake View. It's worth noting that preceding Karl's article was a one-page profile of him. In the profile, Karl mentions having been treated for tuberculosis in Europe in 1926-27. "I did not have to read Thomas Mann's 'The Magic Mountain,' " Karl said. "I saw it. But I also learned that there are no absolutes in tuberculosis treatment."

The short profile ended with the writer – the piece was signed only "W.E.S." – noting of Karl: "On campus Professor Link is known as one of the few free spirits. He shuns barbers and society – but his lectures go unmatched. His favorite composer is Johann Sebastian Bach – 'that's the Lutheran in me.' His ultimate ambition – 'to become a cowboy and live on a ranch 7 miles square. That's the gambler in me. The sum of the digits 214 [his Lake View room number] is 7.'"

Karl's article was lengthy, around 5,000 words. At its heart was this sentence, from the article's middle: "Isolation – isolation

8. The Road to Warfarin

from friends, kith and kin and preoccupation with the irrevocable past are without doubt contributing causes to that muffled unhappiness or frank unhappiness that one sees here at Lake View."

Karl then noted how in Russia health care professionals had experimented successfully with "night sanitoriums" that allowed patients to work or otherwise conduct normal business during the day. And in England and Scotland, there were "village settlements" that allowed patients living there and responding well to treatment to work and be productive.

No doubt Karl's rising prominence as a scientist factored into the reception of "As Seen from 214." The bed linen hit the fan. The *Wisconsin State Journal* put the story above the fold on page one Sunday, April 7, 1946, with this headline: "Lake View Policy Delays Recoveries, Dr. Link Charges." The secondary headline: "Scientist, Ill at Sanitorium, Puts Blame on the Management."

The story opened: "Writing from his bed in Lake View sanitorium for the tubercular, Dr. Karl Paul Link, world-famous scientist, Saturday charged that the management of the sanitorium is creating mental unrest in the patients that is retarding their recovery.

"Patients are held in virtual isolation which contributes to the 'unrest, tension and mental dissolution that one can sense at Lake View,' Dr. Link [wrote]."

There were follow-up newspaper articles, and the state board of health appointed a committee to examine the situation at Lake View. At a meeting of the committee in May 1946, Karl showed up, and, according to a story in the next day's *State Journal*, spent 45 minutes explaining what was wrong at Lake View – and with those who criticized him for voicing his opinion.

"I wrote my way into this medical lion's den," Karl said, "through an article on behalf of the tubercular. I have come here from my bed to defend it."

While all this was percolating – in late April 1946 – Karl was elected to the National Academy of Sciences, a prestigious society established by an act of Congress, signed by President Abraham Lincoln and charged with advising the nation on matters of science and technology. Membership is one of the highest honors an American scientist can receive.

Given his willingness to wade into issues outside his laboratory – on any matter he deemed important – it's no surprise this was not the last time that controversy and accomplishment would engage Karl Paul Link almost simultaneously. His personality made it nearly unavoidable.

Also of import, in late 1945, was the return to Madison of Mark Stahmann, Karl's student who had worked on isolating the hemorrhagic agent in sweet clover – and was on the first dicumarol patent application – and who had gone to New York City to work with Max Bergmann.

We've already seen that Karl reached out to Stahmann when Bergmann died in late 1944, and that Stahmann greatly appreciated Karl's help.

According to Stahmann, his return to Madison was initiated by Karl's illness. In a brief, unpublished memoir that was made available for this narrative by Stahmann's daughter, Dr. Marcia Richards, Stahmann wrote, "I returned to the University of Wisconsin to supervise Dr. Link's laboratory while he was ill and confined to a sanitorium."

In his 1958 New York City lecture on dicumarol, Karl said, "While I was in the sanitorium in 1945-46 the laboratory work was practically at a standstill. There were few students available, since most of them were still in the armed forces."

This apparent discrepancy – Stahmann's claim he was running Karl's lab, and Karl's assertion that the lab was at a standstill – is part of a larger, egregious split between the two men that requires a closer look. Conventional wisdom on the split, such as it exists, centers around the patenting of warfarin, which, as the world now knows, became a hugely successful

8. THE ROAD TO WARFARIN

rodenticide as well as a human anticoagulant. Among its earliest beneficiaries was President Dwight D. Eisenhower.

It was in his 1958 New York City speech that Karl sketched his version of how the 1930s work in his lab to find what was killing cows – which led to the discovery of dicumarol – eventually evolved into an investigation into the compound's potential viability as a rat killer.

In Karl's account, he noted that dating to 1940 and continuing until 1942, two of his students – Ralph Overman and John B. Field – along with Karl's professorial colleague, Carl Baumann, "had studied extensively the action of dicumarol in the laboratory rat, and the effect of the diet on the response, specifically the influence of vitamin K and foods rich in it."

Karl then said – in his New York lecture – that in late 1942 he himself "set up field trials to ascertain the suitability of dicumarol for rodenticidal purpose."

What Karl found, he told his New York audience, was that the activity of dicumarol in rats was not high enough to make it an efficient exterminator, especially since the natural foods available to rats contained vitamin K, which then increased their tolerance for the dicumarol.

Still, his students continued to synthesize coumarins, which, as noted, eventually numbered more than 100. Karl said that numbers 40-65 were synthesized by Miyoshi Ikawa, a doctoral student of Karl's from California.

Ikawa arrived in Madison at the urging of Linus Pauling, his graduate advisor at Caltech, who suggested him to Karl because of negative post-Pearl Harbor Japanese sentiment in California, where Pasadena had been declared a military zone. Karl had to advocate with a variety of authorities to bring Ikawa to Wisconsin. Ikawa later shared a lab at UC-Berkeley with Emil Fischer's son, eventually moving to the University of New Hampshire, where he spent most of his career.

When Karl was institutionalized at Lake View, from late 1945 to April 1946, he said he "kept the aged tuberculosis out of my mind by studying laboratory records and reading the history of rodent control from ancient to modern times."

This description is backed up by the recollection of William H. Stone, a young student of Karl's who went onto a distinguished career in genetics.

Stone's recollection: "I recall visiting Dr. Link at a sanatorium in Madison where he was being treated for tuberculosis. He was sitting up in his bed as I entered his private room."

Before Stone could even muster a greeting, he recalled Karl saying, "Bill, I had a dream last night that warfarin would be a very efficient rat poison."

Now, it should be noted that Karl could not at that time have said exactly that – he hadn't minted the word "warfarin" yet. But Stone's recollection is specific enough to remember that their conversation continued into whether rats might eventually become resistant to the effects of the drug.

When Karl left the sanitorium in spring 1946, it coincided with the return from military service of his student Lester Scheel, to whom, Karl said, he assigned "the task of reappraising the anticoagulant activity" of compounds 40-65.

"In 1946-48," Karl said in his 1958 New York talk, "he [Scheel] defined coumarins numbers 42 and 63 as being much more potent than dicumarol in the rat and the dog, as capable of producing a more uniform anticoagulant response, and as having the quality of maintaining a more severe state of hypothrombinemia [leading to internal bleeding] without inducing visible bleeding."

Karl said that in early 1948 he told Scheel and another student, Dorothy Wu, "that I wanted to propose [synthesized coumarin] number 42 for rodenticidal use."

The reaction, Karl said, bordered on disbelief.

"This proposal shook the laboratory," Karl told the New York audience. "I can sum up by stating the consensus opinion 'the boss has really gone off the deep end this time.'"

8. The Road to Warfarin

(One student who was in Karl's lab in 1946-48, Clint Ballou, recalled that a scientific paper published around this time in England – promoting the possibility of dicumarol as a rodenticide – hastened Karl's desire to find another more potent coumarin that would perform the task. "I remember," Ballou noted, "Link storming into the lab one morning shouting, 'We can't let them make dicumarol into a rat poison. The M.D.s will never touch it again.'")

Karl ended that portion of his New York talk with this: "To make a long story very short, early in 1948 number 42 was promoted for rodent control under the auspices of the Wisconsin Alumni Research Foundation through the able, enthusiastic, and public-spirited Ward Ross, general manager of the organization. Within a short time this effort revolutionized the art of rodent control, (multiple doses as opposed to the single dose of highly toxic poisons), and warfarin quickly became and still is the leader in the rodenticide field."

Karl concluded, "The name warfarin was coined by me by combining the first letters of the Wisconsin Alumni Research Foundation with the 'arin' from coumarin – and it is now a household word throughout the world."

In hindsight, one name is conspicuous in its absence from Karl's account: Mark Stahmann.

Stahmann's version of the events from 1942-48 is, unsurprisingly, quite different.

It is contained in two letters totaling 27 pages written by Stahmann on February 19-20, 1951 to the WARF board of trustees, and the attention of George Haight, president of the trustees.

At the outset, Stahmann noted that "this letter is to review my contributions to the invention covered in [the Warfarin patent] issued on September 16, 1947 to Mark A. Stahmann, Miyoshi Ikawa and Karl Paul Link."

The letter goes onto describe what Stahmann believes were his contributions to the invention and what he feels were Karl's efforts to negate those contributions.

Before examining Stahmann's letter in more detail, it's worth noting that if Karl did indeed try to minimize Stahmann's involvement, it would have been out of character.

Early in his professional life, in Scotland, Karl had experienced a superior, J.C. Irvine, whom Karl felt took credit for work that he, Karl, had performed. It left a mark – nearly torpedoing Karl's nascent career – and casts doubt on the likelihood Karl would engage in the practice himself. Indeed, there is abundant testimony that the opposite was true, and that Karl was open to sharing credit.

Earlier in this narrative the student who with Stahmann originally isolated the hemorrhagic agent in spoiled sweet clover, Harold Campbell, is quoted talking about Karl's generosity as a mentor, his insistence that a student find his own way in the lab, a mindset that Campbell said led to more creative results.

In the early 1960s "Men and Molecules" radio program devoted to dicumarol, George Wakerlin, the medical director of the American Heart Association, said this:

"One of the things I was impressed with in our conversations at the University Club in Chicago back in 1945 was the fact Dr. Link was very careful to give due credit to the members of his research team. When there were differences, he accepted the viewpoint of his younger men, and they would go back into the laboratory to determine who was right and who was wrong. It seems to me that Dr. Link said his younger men were sometimes right, he was sometimes right, and he was sometimes wrong."

In that same radio program, Karl said, "A captain of a ship doesn't do anything except stay with the ship, no matter what happens. I can honestly say that as the project operator, we operated pretty closely as a little commune. Very seldom did I prevent any of these workers from trying out a hunch they had, unless it was really way off beat."

Karl concluded, "In a general way, they did the work, I did the directing."

8. THE ROAD TO WARFARIN

In a eulogy after Karl's death, his student Saul Roseman, who later became chairman of the biology department at Johns Hopkins University, spoke about the "special affinity" Karl enjoyed with his students. Roseman quoted yet another student, Fred Kummerow: "Karl Paul was the champion of many graduate students... and we were all grateful for his willingness to take our cause as his own."

And another student, Charlie Huebner: "He made us all part of his family, personally as well as scientifically. I have since noticed that very few, if any, professors give more than a minimum of passing interest in the development and the education of their students. We didn't realize how specifically fortunate we were. The mechanics and small details of research can be taught by many but few could teach the spirit, joy and excitement of research like he could. These were the really important things I learned from him."

It is also worth noting, before examining Stahmann's contention that Karl claimed credit that Stahmann was due, how Karl chose to close his celebrated 1944 Harvey lecture in New York City on the discovery of dicumarol:

"And now in closing I wish to emphasize that what has been presented tonight is not an individual achievement," Karl said. "It is the creation of a loyal, hard-working band of research students, against whom at times the pendulum of ill-luck swung heavily. It should be made clear that I did not put up any of the pillars or flying buttresses of the edifice. I merely attended to some of the general architectonic features and bridge work. But it is my good lot to be the spokesman – the reporter – for those who made the discoveries. Let me tell you the secret of their success. They brought to this study but one working hypothesis – that it could be done; but one philosophy – that there is no defeat except giving up trying. As servants of a great commonwealth they had ever before them hope that they might through this work contribute to the welfare of mankind."

Now, to Stahmann.

In Stahmann's 1951 letter to the WARF trustees regarding warfarin, he notes that after he left Madison to join Bergmann in New York City in 1942, he continued to work on anticoagulants. Ikawa, meanwhile, was involved in similar work in Madison. According to Stahmann, on Oct. 20, 1943, Karl sent to Stahmann for approval a manuscript summarizing the anticoagulant activity of the new coumarin compounds. A paper "incorporating data from both Mr. Ikawa and my reports [Stahmann wrote] was published in June 1944."

The paper listed as authors M. Ikawa, M.A. Stahmann and K.P. Link. The June 1944 date is important because under United States law a patent must be filed within a year of the first public disclosure or it loses its patentability.

In his 1951 letter, Stahmann claims that he was responsible for keeping that one-year window for patenting the new anticoagulant coumarins and the process of making them front and center in discussions and letters over the ensuing months.

Stahmann mentioned a dicumarol conference in Chicago that he attended in late January 1945. "The question of patenting [the new anticoagulant coumarins] was not then discussed," Stahmann wrote.

He continued: "After this conference, I visited Madison [Stahmann was still living on the East Coast] to discuss an offer which had been made to me for a staff position in the [UW] Biochemistry Department and while there I again urged Dr. Link that this patent be written. On my return trip I made a special stop in Chicago to recommend to [WARF managing director Ward] Ross that this patent be written. I did this because eight of the 12 months in which we could legally file an application had already passed with no action being taken toward patent application."

A few days later, having returned to the East Coast, Stahmann wrote a letter to Ross and George Schley, an Indianapolis-based attorney retained by WARF to assist in patent cases, again pointing out the urgency of making the patent filing by spring.

8. The Road to Warfarin

According to Stahmann, Ross wrote back: "I discussed briefly over the telephone with Mr. Schley last week the matter of the proposed new [patent]. He is going to make an effort to do something about this case before he leaves for the West on March 3. In any event he has my authorization to proceed."

By late February 1945, Schley was ready to pull the trigger and file a patent application for the new coumarin compounds and the process of making them. As we will see, the question of who should be credited as "inventors" on the patent came up. Decades later, some assume it was this question, and its resolution, that caused the rupture of the relationship between Karl and Stahmann. Perhaps – but if so, it took some time to surface.

Part of the relevant material – letters cited by Stahmann in his 1951 27-page memo to the WARF trustees – was provided to the author by Stahmann's daughter, who kept material related to her dad in boxes in the basement of her home outside Milwaukee. It should be noted that in quoting Stahmann's 27-page memo, this author has not examined all the original letters Stahmann cites.

So, to the 1945 patent application.

On February 22, 1945, according to Stahmann, Schley, the patent attorney, wrote to Ross, the WARF managing director, about the proposed patent.

"Who are the inventors?" Schley asked.

The attorney then lays out four possible choices for "the inventive entity." The names included Stahmann, who continued to work on the anticoagulant compounds after leaving Madison for the Rockefeller Institute; Ikawa, who picked up the work in Madison after Stahmann departed; and Karl Paul Link, director of the lab that originated and conducted the research. It should be remembered that all three names were listed as authors of the April and June 1944 papers that, when published, began the 12-month window for a patent application.

Now Schley listed the inventor choices:

"a. Stahmann alone.
"b. Stahmann and Ikawa.

"c. Stahmann and Link.
"d. Stahmann, Ikawa and Link."

Schley told Ross: "I am inclined to file the application in the name of the three men. And then if we find we are wrong, we can drop one or two, but if we have too few to start with we can't add. Do you agree?"

Presumably, Ross concurred, because two days later, according to Stahmann, Schley telephoned Stahmann in New York and discussed the options and their preference for listing all three names. (It should be noted that by most accounts it would have been unusual not to list the names of all three authors of the paper a year earlier as inventors; and it would have been equally unusual not to have Karl, who directed the lab where most of the work was done, as an inventor in any case.)

Stahmann said he sent Schley a telegram later that day: FAVOR FILING WITH THREE NAMES."

In his 1951 memo, Stahmann notes that he later regretted sending that wire.

"My decision to include Link in this application," Stahmann wrote [not that it was his decision to make], "was made without adequate thought and was influenced by Mr. Schley's advice that a name could be dropped later and that it might strengthen the patent if he were included. Furthermore, I had then just accepted a position in the Biochemistry Department and feared that if Link were not included he might block my work and advancement."

That was how Stahmann viewed it in hindsight, in 1951.

Two other letters written in February 1945 – and cited by Stahmann in the 1951 memo – are worth considering.

In a Feb. 5 letter to Schley, the patent attorney, Stahmann referenced his work on the compound while he was based in New York, as well as a 1943 report he wrote describing it.

"Since my report was written," Stahmann noted, "Mr. Ikawa and Dr. Link have done considerable work on [the compound]. The results of all our work were published in [the April and June 1944 papers]."

8. The Road to Warfarin

So Stahmann, in February 1945, gave Karl (and Ikawa) credit for their work on the compound.

Another letter quoted by Stahmann in his 1951 memo – again, the actual letter has not been seen by this author – is from Karl to Ward Ross, WARF managing director. It was written Feb. 13, 1945 and concerns Compound 42, its patent potential, and the inventors.

"The question is," Karl wrote, "should the Foundation [WARF] file a patent… It is my personal opinion that the Foundation has nothing to lose by attempting to patent… whether or not it might gain anything thereby is questionable…

"In my opinion the inventors in this case are Stahmann and Ikawa – I was in constant touch with the work but I don't see how anything that I did contributed to the inventive concepts involved."

That was a seemingly magnanimous stance for Karl to take, especially in that the director of a lab would generally be included on the list of inventors of discoveries made in his lab, as, indeed, Karl was when the patent was filed in April 1945.

Another preeminent UW scientist-researcher of later vintage, Hector DeLuca, who worked closely with Harry Steenbock and took classes on campus from Karl, said it would have been highly unusual to omit Karl from the list of inventors. "He set up the lab," DeLuca said, in an interview for this book. "It's his lab. He hired Stahmann. He's part of the discovery no matter how you turn it. You can't take him out."

At the time – February 1945 – Karl was still months from entering the sanitorium, where, he later said, he began to think about the possibility of the anticoagulant coumarins as a rodenticide – and presumably the commercial possibilities that would make it important to patent.

In the meantime, Stahmann did the legwork to get the patent application filed. In late February 1945 he flew to Indianapolis and helped attorney Schley frame the application. The patent application was filed April 2, 1945.

In his 1951 memo, Stahmann wrote that in February 1945 he had accepted an offer to return to Madison to join the Biochemistry Department once the war ended. Other accounts (including one from Stahmann) state his return to Madison, in the fall of 1945, was at Karl's behest – to run Karl's lab while he was being treated for tuberculosis. (It's possible Stahmann moved up his return to take over Karl's lab.)

In an essay for the 1982 book, *The New Frontiers in Plant Biochemistry*, Stahmann wrote, "I was asked to return to Madison in the fall of 1945 to take charge of Link's laboratory while he was in a sanitorium recovering from tuberculosis."

Karl stated it was while in the sanitorium that he began research on rodenticides and began to envision the possibility of the anticoagulant coumarins – the patent had yet to be granted – as a rat poison.

Meanwhile, Stahmann was in Karl's lab, doing assays – Stahmann wrote in his 1982 essay – on mice and learning that one of the coumarins – number 42 – was extremely toxic to them, 100-200 times as toxic as dicumarol.

"My work had clearly shown that [Compound 42] would be a [highly effective rodenticide]," Stahmann wrote.

His research angered Karl, according to Stahmann.

"Link left the sanitorium against the doctor's advice and told me and our chairman that he alone wanted to continue [the lab work with anticoagulants] ... [Link] forced me out of his laboratory and said that I should find other work."

Stahmann's account is problematic. As noted previously in this narrative, immediately before and after Karl's departure from Lake View in April 1946, he was preoccupied with conditions there, to the point of writing a controversial article, giving press interviews and appearing at a hearing. Further, he does not seem to have left the sanitorium against doctor's orders. An early April *State Journal* article on the sanitorium controversy stated Karl "expects to return to his home in Madison this month with the arresting of the progress of his case of tuberculosis." Less than two weeks later, Karl was back home in the Highlands.

8. The Road to Warfarin

Still, something caused a significant rupture in the relationship between Link and Stahmann. It's evident from Link's erasing Stahmann whenever Karl recalled the history of the development of dicumarol and warfarin. One might argue the extent of Stahmann's involvement, but clearly he was a figure of some importance. It's evident, too, in Stahmann's later bitterness when asked about Link, to the point of trying to cast doubt on one of Karl's favorite stories, about the farmer Ed Carlson bringing the dead cow and a bucket of cow's blood to Madison in the early 1930s, which led to Link's anticoagulant work.

After Karl's death in 1978, Robert Burris, preparing a biographical essay on Karl for the National Academies Press, asked Stahmann, among others, for input. Stahmann's comments to Burris were highly negative and included this: "I still think [the bucket of blood story] is fiction and that it should not be published as a true story. I suggest you delete this fable. Perhaps we should check to see if an Ed Carlson ever lived in the Deer Park vicinity and lost a heifer from the hemorrhagic sweet clover disease."

As research for this book showed, it was not fiction.

What lay behind the break? Perhaps it wasn't any single episode or point of contention, but rather was cumulative – a mix of ego skirmishes, credit disputes and other disagreements, including but not limited to the patenting of the new coumarin compounds and subsequent research on them as a possible rodenticide, that finally became combustible. Did Stahmann overreach? Did Karl feel threatened? In any case, the fuse burned slowly.

Karl returned to his lab from the sanitorium in spring 1946. He may not have been pleased with the work Stahmann had done with anticoagulants in his absence, but the patent applied for in 1945 was granted – with, it appears, very little fanfare – on Sept. 16, 1947. As noted, Stahmann, Ikawa and Link were all named as inventors on the patent, the first sentence of which reads:

> *"Our invention relates to certain new 3-substituted 4-hydroxycoumarins, which have anticoagulant properties; and to the process of making them."*

What appears likely is that while Link's lab continued to work on the anticoagulants from 1946-48 – the reader will recall he credited his student Lester Scheel with recognizing compound numbers 42 and 63 as being especially potent, which led Karl to envision them as a rodenticide – so, too, did Stahmann work on the anticoagulants in this period, outside Karl's lab. Did Karl know and would he have approved? As we will soon see, Karl cites certain unspecified "agreements" that make it appear he did not and would not.

But prior, in early 1948, Karl assisted in Stahmann's effort to secure a position at Northwestern University. This may not have been wholly altruistic on Karl's part, as success would remove Stahmann from Madison. The position was head of the biochemistry unit of Northwestern's Rheumatic Fever Research Institute.

On Feb. 18, Dr. Alvin F. Coburn, founder and director of the institute, wrote to Karl: "Thank you so much for your... biographical sketch of Mark Stahmann. Mark was here Monday and everybody here, including Dean Miller, reacted just as I did. Briefly, we want Mark to head up the biochemical work of our group."

Coburn continued, "Once again I want you to know that we appreciate the generous assistance which you have given to us."

The same day, Coburn wrote Stahmann: "We feel that you are the perfect person to have in our biochemistry unit... We offer you a salary of $9,000 per annum; equipment, supplies and whatever funds you feel reasonable for technical assistants."

Two months later, in April 1948, with Stahmann considering the Northwestern position (and Northwestern, as we shall see, assuming he had accepted it for the coming fall), a Biochemistry Department staff meeting was held in Madison, apparently to discuss how much of an effort should be made to retain Stahmann. Minutes of the meeting – signed by Conrad Elvehjem, the department chairman – are in Karl's UW archive.

Karl was present but did actively participate in the discussion. Elvehjem noted: "Dr. Link indicated he wished to remain neutral in the matter. He presented the material which he had sent to Northwestern University regarding Dr. Stahmann's consideration there. He did not wish to make any specific recommendation regarding Dr. Stahmann's ability to direct research work."

On Sept. 30, 1948, Elvehjem wrote a letter to Ira Baldwin, Dean of the College of Agriculture, that began, "As I have already indicated to you, Dr. Mark Stahmann has decided that he would like to stay at the University of Wisconsin."

Elvehjem notes that "the staff" felt "that Dr. Stahmann would be better off if he went to a new environment where he could carry on his work free from the difficulties which have arisen at Wisconsin." Stahmann's teaching duties for fall, Elvehjem noted, had already been reassigned.

But Elvehjem concluded, "In spite of these facts the department definitely recognizes his ability in research and on this basis the department is willing to cooperate in efforts to retain him."

Stahmann was staying in Madison.

Coburn, from Northwestern, wrote to Karl on October 6:

"Dear Karl:
"Our team is preparing for the kick-off but must go through the first game without a center. I had regarded Mark as the roving center. We had completed his laboratory, rented a house for him in Evanston and had his first month's salary check waiting for him. Conditions beyond our control kept Mark in Madison."

Karl, we may be sure, was not pleased. His outgoing correspondence from this time on this issue does not survive, but in his archive are letters from colleagues around the country expressing dismay at the situation. One noted: "The news about Stahmann was distressing, but no surprise."

On Nov. 21, future Nobel laureate Stanford Moore wrote Karl from New York City: "I feel sorry for Mark, but he certainly got himself and his friends into a mess. I hope that Mark and his wife realize the seriousness of the mistakes, because only if they do can they correct their behavior in the future. I trust they are young enough and flexible enough to profit by their mistakes, although I sometimes wonder whether Mark will ever mature sufficiently to know how to handle himself."

With Stahmann remaining in Madison, it was perhaps inevitable that the simmering tension between Stahmann and Karl would boil over.

In early July 1949, Karl wrote a letter to Conrad Elvehjem, chairman of the Biochemistry Department. Karl had apparently just learned the extent of Stahmann's 1946-1948 anticoagulant work and papers prepared describing it.

"I attempted," Karl wrote, "to get Stahmann to see that he was violating agreements made, whereupon he replied that he was out to get me by any method and to protect his rights. He took a pass at me and I can say that only a charitable heart kept me from pulping his face. I insist on a hearing to renew all agreements made. My generosity toward him died this afternoon...."

"If necessary," Karl wrote Elvehjem, "I shall take legal action against Stahmann and any administrator who OKs publication of results by Stahmann in violation of agreements made."

Around the same time, Stahmann wrote his own letter to university administrators, about another meeting, claiming it was Karl who provoked a physical altercation.

In Stahmann's later letter to the WARF trustees, he claimed that his work "clearly pointed to the commercial utility of [the new compounds] as a rodenticide," noting they had "an unexpected high toxicity in mice."

In the letter – written after Compound 42 had become famous as warfarin – Stahmann notes that he stepped away from

8. The Road to Warfarin

further anticoagulant research [after 1948] as "I considered [it] Dr. Link's field of research. Instead, Dr. Link's group continued the study with rats."

The two had very little to do with one another after summer 1949. Publicly, the feud – unknown outside the Biochemistry Department – bubbled up one more time, upon publication of a *Reader's Digest* article on warfarin in March 1951, in which Stahmann's involvement in its development and patenting – however large or small that involvement may have been – was never mentioned. But that was it.

Karl's career was in ascendance – in 1951, he was nominated for the prestigious Hoblitzelle Agricultural Award; the following year he won the Cameron prize in Scotland; and before the decade was out, he would twice be awarded the Lasker, a top science honor that often precedes the awarding of the Nobel Prize. Stahmann's subsequent career was much less celebrated, but accomplished, nonetheless. He remained at UW-Madison. He earned a Guggenheim Fellowship and a Fulbright Scholarship.

After Karl's death in 1978, when asked for comment by Robert Burris for a biographical essay, Stahmann (who died in 2000) was, as noted earlier, still bitter. Yet he also wrote Burris this: "For most of the time when I was a graduate student and while I was running his laboratory for him as a staff member, [Link] treated me very well. He often invited me to his home for dinners or parties with his friends. He loaned me the use of his second old car. I appreciated this and had the dents taken out of its fenders."

9. RATTOR

THE FIRST PUBLIC INDICATION that something big was again brewing in the lab of Karl Paul Link on the University of Wisconsin campus came on a Tuesday afternoon in March 1949.

Carl H. Krieger, director of general laboratories for WARF, addressed a March 29 meeting of the Wisconsin Pest Control Operators Association at the Hotel Loraine in downtown Madison. A *Wisconsin State Journal* reporter, John Newhouse, soon to be a favorite of Karl's, was in attendance.

Newhouse's front-page story in the next day's paper was headlined: "UW Comes Up With a Deadly Rat-Killer." The article was accompanied by a photo of the students Dorothy Wu and Lester Scheel, "working in the laboratory of Karl Paul Link."

Newhouse wrote, "Known as Compound 42, the new rat killer holds the promise of wiping out rat colonies completely, rather than – as with other poisons – wiping out a few and leaving the rest to their age-old role of depredation. Against the new killer, the cunning of the rat is of no avail. He can't taste the new killer. He can't smell the new killer. And it has the further great advantage that it is slow acting."

Newhouse reached out to Karl, who is quoted in the story recalling how years earlier, in 1942, rabbits given dicumarol hemorrhaged and died. Karl remembered saying, "Ought to check it for an exterminating agent." But at the time, the focus was on developing a human anticoagulant.

Two years later, Karl said, one of his lab assistants, Lloyd Graf, learned that a derivative of the drug was killing rats. Karl urged Graf to continue his work, but two days later, Graf was called into the Navy.

9. RATTOR

Then, in 1948, a scientific paper from England, published by J. A. O'Connor, made the case for dicumarol as a rodenticide. As noted previously in this narrative, this troubled Karl for two reasons: He knew that the diet of rodents contained enough vitamin K to counteract the bleeding from dicumarol; more urgently, Karl could foresee nothing good coming from conflating a human heart medicine with a rat poison. He told Newhouse he made a pronouncement in the lab: "We better figure out a better rat killer, quick."

They thought they had it in Compound 42, and they were right. Things came together quickly. The patent had been secured a year earlier (1947), and by 1949, tests were being conducted that would yield approval for its sale to consumers.

A later UW News Service release noted: "Several hundred field tests, carried out in a nationwide testing program in September 1949, have demonstrated the outstanding effectiveness of Warfarin [the name was adopted in early 1950] rodenticides in killing rats and mice.

"These were conducted under an experimental permit issued by the production and marketing administration of the U.S. Department of Agriculture at that time. Between 85 and 90 percent of all tests show complete or satisfactory results. Tests were carried on by the wildlife service of the U.S. Department of the Interior, the U.S. Public Health Service, city and state health departments, professional exterminators, and individual farmers and householders."

Karl, one shouldn't be surprised to learn, got in the act himself. The Sunday, December 4, 1949, *Wisconsin State Journal* contained a full-page feature on Compound 42, headlined, "Murder – For Rats."

The story, written by Newhouse, the reporter who had first introduced Compound 42 to readers nine months earlier, featured two area farmers who had read about the compound in the *State Journal*, contacted Karl, and had success using it. At the bottom of the page was a photograph of Karl at home in the Highlands

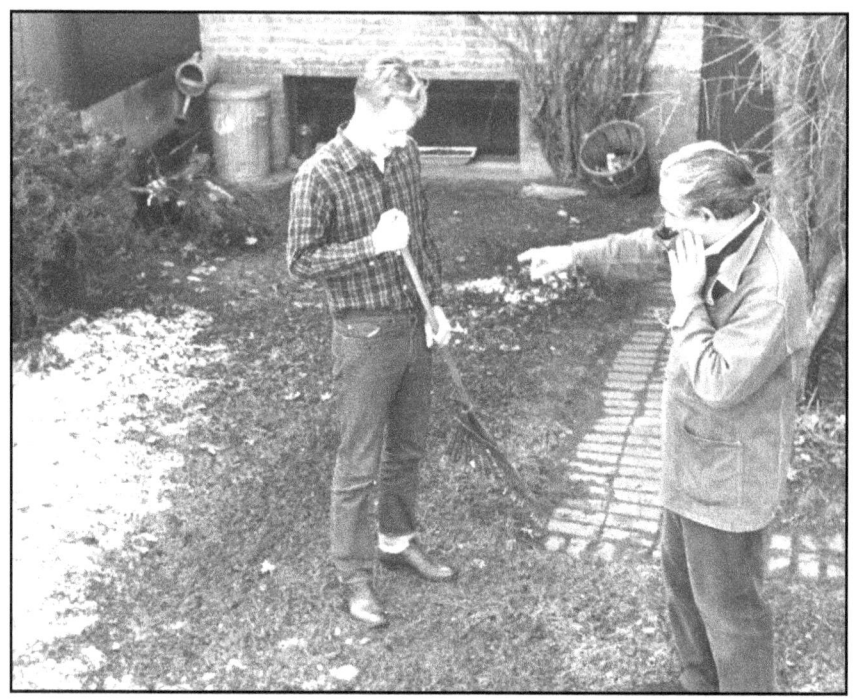

Karl and his second son, Tom. (Link family)

with a homemade coop he used for chickens on which he was testing Compound 42. The chickens – along with pets and other domestic animals – were unharmed by Compound 42. The photo cutline noted: "Dr. Link had some of the chickens for dinner."

In a campus talk on the 75th anniversary of Karl beginning his anticoagulant work, Karl's son, Tom Link, recalled the chickens.

"I must have been 10 or 11 and we had these cages in the yard," Tom said. "They were six [feet] by 10 [feet], with wheels, and there were all these chickens in them. He was feeding the chickens. It was my job to make sure the chickens were moved. The chickens would eat up all the grass within a matter of a few hours. Once they were full grown, they were shipped off to a slaughterhouse on Pheasant Branch Road in Middleton, and of course we ate them."

9. RATTOR

Tom concluded, "What I didn't know was he was trying to kill them with warfarin."

A week after the chicken story, in a "society" column in the *State Journal*, it was reported that Karl was now referring to himself as the "Rattor," a designation he would keep for the remainder of his life.

Warfarin went on the market for consumers in June 1950. Over the next many months, it received a staggering amount of coverage in newspapers and magazines across the country. Scores of newspaper headlines – "New Rat Killer Now on Market," "New Rat Poison May Eliminate All Rodents, "Sad Days Ahead for Rats" – shouted the news.

Karl was more celebrated than ever, but he was not slowing down. Just the opposite.

"Link promoted warfarin as a rodenticide very actively himself," UW biochemist Dave Nelson said. "He was out there pitching with the farmers and legislators. Developing simple, cheap, effective methods of exposing animals to the bait. I think in this sense he was a perfect example of a scientist who really took the Wisconsin Idea charge seriously. He went out there and did what the state paid him to do. He helped a lot of farmers learn how to use this compound and saved a lot of crops."

According to a January 1951 article – by his now-favorite chronicler, John Newhouse – Karl quickly, in summer 1950, established a relationship with numerous Dane County farmers in order to improve and perfect his rat poison.

"If this new poison is going to work," Karl told Newhouse, in an article published in the *State Journal* January 28, 1951, "it's got to kill rats under the most difficult conditions. And that means going out to the farms themselves to try it out."

Tom Link remembers accompanying his father – and reporter Newhouse – on a trip to a farm on Highway 14 in Cross Plains. It was likely January 1951. "The coldest day I ever experienced," Tom recalled.

Never let it be said Karl was averse to getting out in the elements.

Driving "a well-worn station wagon," Newhouse wrote, "a rolling laboratory for the war on the rat," Karl enlisted nine farmers to the cause.

"Link's poison is now being used the country over," Newhouse wrote. "His current experiments involve refinements of poisoning."

Beginning on July 18, 1950, Karl mixed the poison and set the baits at the farms. He visited at least one of the farms for 51 consecutive days, putting 2,600 miles on his car. The farmers got used to seeing him but one night at dusk he was pursuing a weakened rat around a corner of a barn and a law officer leveled a gun at him. Another time, a farm hand asked him to pull a tooth, and Karl obliged. Field work occasionally engaged his sense of the absurd.

It was a heady time – widespread acclaim, with more challenging and rewarding work ahead. And yet. Less than two weeks after the publication of the Newhouse story on Karl's Dane County farm experiments, a new controversy erupted. Unlike the quarrel involving Mark Stahmann, this one played out across the front pages of Madison's newspapers. And it involved not a former student of Karl's, but rather a UW scientist with a towering reputation equal to Karl's – Harry Steenbock.

The February 9, 1951, topline headline in *The Capital Times* read: "Link Charges His Work 'Sabotaged' By Dr. Steenbock."

A secondary headline read: "Declares Discoverer of Vitamin D Kept New Aspirin Off Market."

The *Cap Times* article was written by "John Hunter," a byline that would eventually be changed to John Patrick Hunter, which became a well-known name in Wisconsin journalism.

Hunter's story began, "Prof. Karl Paul Link, university faculty member and one of the nation's top biochemists, charged Thursday night that his scientific work is being 'sabotaged' by Dr. Harry Steenbock, one of the founders of the Wisconsin

9. RATTOR

Alumni Research Foundation (WARF), and the discoverer of vitamin D irradiation.

"Prof. Link made the charge in a public address before 250 persons in the university biochemistry building, and elaborated on his statements in an interview with *The Capital Times* today.

"Both Prof. Link and Dr. Steenbock are nationally known scientists.

"Link charged that Steenbock attempted to pass judgment on his discoveries and his inventions which 'he (Steenbock) is scientifically incapable of doing.'"

Karl told the paper: "I am fed up with seeing administration and staff members crawl like worms before the Steenbock dollar."

Over the next several days, a series of articles in *The Capital Times*, *Wisconsin State Journal*, and *The Daily Cardinal* traced Karl's ire to a meeting of the WARF Board of Trustees at the Madison Club a few years earlier. At that meeting, Karl said, Steenbock had used his clout to convince the board not to allow one of Karl's inventions – a safer form of aspirin that reduced the risk of hemorrhage – to be sold over the counter rather than prescription only. Additionally, Karl charged, Steenbock had blocked Karl's efforts to see that laboratory workers shared in the profits of patented inventions.

In truth, the uneasy relationship between Link and Steenbock traced back at least a decade, and likely farther. Their personalities could hardly have been less similar. In broad strokes, Steenbock was a play-it-by-the-book and keep-the-lid-on type of character, while Karl was willing to play a hunch, double down, and do it all in public.

In 1942, at a meeting of the Biochemistry Department on campus, the two had disagreed on the future leadership of plant physiology in the department, with Steenbock promoting his right-hand man, Forrest Quackenbush, and Karl sticking behind the scientist who had mentored him, William Tottingham.

According to a March 6, 1942 letter, written by Steenbock to department Dean Chris Christensen, Karl had approached Steenbock in the hall after the meeting. Words were exchanged, and then, according to Steenbock, Karl "stepped up to me with an oath, placed both hands at my throat and threatened to knock me down."

Over the years, others have placed this exchange as starting in the Biochemistry men's room and spilling out into the hall. Henry Lardy, who earned two graduate degrees at UW-Madison in the 1940s and then joined the faculty of the University's Enzyme Institute, claimed he was present for that one.

"I happened to be the only guy who witnessed the battle between Steenbock and Link in the men's john," Lardy told the UW Oral History Program. "I don't know just who said what, but I happened to be in the toilet at the time. Steenbock and Link happened to accidentally come in, or one was in and the other accidentally came in. The argument started getting hotter and hotter, and I quickly got out of there."

No matter the number or location of confrontations, one thing is clear: There was no love lost between Link and Steenbock.

Hector DeLuca came to UW-Madison as a graduate student in 1951, just as the Link-Steenbock feud was spilling over into the newspapers. DeLuca was a rising star and had received a personal letter from Steenbock inviting him to work and study in his lab in Madison.

"To me," DeLuca said, in an interview for this book, "that was not an offer, it was a command." Such was Steenbock's prestige.

DeLuca, who eventually inherited Steenbock's lab, served as chairman of the Biochemistry Department and produced numerous patentable discoveries in a celebrated career, said he got along well with Karl, despite the fractured Link-Steenbock relationship.

9. RATTOR

"Steenbock refused to talk about Karl Paul Link," DeLuca said.

DeLuca recalled that as a grad student, he had a one-on-one seminar scheduled with Karl.

"I got up to speak," DeLuca said, "and he said, 'Sit down. I am talking today. You're not.' And he talked about something political – something related to Russia. He was hilarious. He sat down, put up his feet and said, 'You see these boots? These are hobnail boots. And they're made in Russia.' I never did give the seminar, but he gave me a good mark.

"I took carbohydrate chemistry from him," DeLuca continued. "He was a world-renowned carbohydrate chemist. I was really looking forward to this. The first half of the class was political. He never said anything about chemistry! But when he did get into the chemistry, he was really good. He knew what he was talking about and he conveyed it in a very interesting and convincing fashion. He was a good speaker and a good teacher, no question about it."

Once DeLuca joined the faculty, he was amused by Karl's flamboyance. "He'd come in the morning, usually around 9:00," DeLuca said. "He'd use the elevator, which was right next to Steenbock's third-floor lab. Karl would use the elevator. He'd come out pulling a little red wagon that had his briefcase in it. In the other hand was a leash with his dog. He loved showing off, he loved attention."

The new aspirin – the source of the 1951 clash between Steenbock and Link – had its own interesting history. It dated to the discovery of the hemorrhagic agent in spoiled sweet clover, which as we know led to the anticoagulant dicumarol. One of the principal components of the H.A. was salicylic acid. It is also the active ingredient in aspirin. Karl reasoned that there might well be anti-clotting elements in aspirin.

Karl later told the *Milwaukee Journal* that his first experiment to test the hypothesis was conducted on a woman in the Link household.

The *Journal* wrote: "A maid in the home was subject to frequent nosebleeds. He [Karl] questioned her and found that she was troubled with recurring headaches and took huge doses of aspirin. Link suggested that she eliminate the aspirin. The nosebleeds ceased."

Karl then turned to another test subject – himself.

"Although Link never uses aspirin as a pain killer," the *Journal* wrote, "he acted as his own guinea pig in his experiments to determine the effect of aspirin on human blood. He took aspirin tablets week after week, and tests of his blood revealed that only four to six five-grain tablets were necessary to make his blood clot more slowly.

"He raised the dose to 8, 10 and then to 12 tablets, dissolved in a glass of milk and taken within 15 minutes of one another."

Karl told the paper: "Ten hours after I had taken 12 tablets the assistant who tested my blood thought I was going to hemorrhage, the clotting took so long."

As noted earlier in this narrative, Karl and his team had worked long and hard during the first half of the 1940s to publicize – and legitimize – what they believed they'd proved about the ability of vitamin K to control hemorrhaging.

They did it first to allay fears that dicumarol could be dangerous. Now Karl envisioned an aspirin that, when combined with a small amount of vitamin K, could still offer pain relief while minimizing risk for those who needed large aspirin doses, including arthritis and rheumatic fever patients.

Karl's new aspirin was patented in September 1945. The *Milwaukee Journal* article appeared the next year, along with a piece in the *Wisconsin State Journal* that said WARF, to which Karl had assigned the patent, had licensed its first commercial use to Lakeside Laboratories of Milwaukee, which marketed it under the trade name Menacyl.

In October 1948, the WARF Board of Trustees met at the Madison Club. It was at that meeting, Karl said, that Harry Steenbock spoke out against selling the vitamin K-infused aspirin over the counter. As a result, Karl said, people were paying "four

9. RATTOR

or five dollars for something that should be available for practically nothing."

As noted, Karl went public with his grievance in an address at the Biochemistry building on February 8, 1951, and in subsequent newspaper interviews. Reporters also reached out to Steenbock.

Steenbock told *The Capital Times*, "I do not even remember attending a meeting and speaking in opposition to Professor Link's aspirin discovery."

Yet in the same article, the *Cap Times* reached out to Ward Ross, WARF managing director – and he sided with Karl.

"Dr. Steenbock spoke to the foundation's board of trustees concerning Link's aspirin discovery," Ross said. "The gist of his remarks was that he was against the proposal to license the product for public sale."

Ross made another remarkable statement that spoke to the power seemingly accorded Steenbock – "the trustees are afraid of him," Karl said – in matters concerning WARF.

"This may cost me my job," Ross said, referring to his rebuttal of Steenbock. "But I am not going to run out on Karl now."

Ross added, "You can quote me as saying it's a mess. I would give anything if it hadn't happened."

In short order – by the following month, March 1951 – the controversy with Steenbock had, at least in Karl's view, conflated with the much less public skirmish involving the origins of warfarin.

The March 1951 issue of the highly popular *Reader's Digest* magazine included an article titled, "Sure Death to Rats." It was written by Paul de Kruif, a longtime contributor to the magazine who was himself a bacteriologist, having developed a successful treatment for syphilis prior to the discovery of penicillin. De Kruif was also a bestselling author – his "Microbe Hunters" sold more than one million copies and was translated into 18 languages – well-known enough that a local Madison newspaper noted when he was in town the previous fall researching his story on rats.

"Through the centuries man has never been able to win the fight against rats," de Kruif wrote early in his piece. "But now Dr. Karl Paul Link of the University of Wisconsin has cooked up a curious chemical poison, called warfarin, which can seal the rodent's doom."

The article related the now familiar story from spoiled sweet clover hay to "Compound 42" to warfarin. Karl got the name, de Kruif noted, by combining WARF and coumarin, the chemical base of dicumarol.

The story credited Miyoshi Ikawa with synthesizing Compound 42. Karl's students Lester Scheel and Dorothy Wu were credited with "working up all the evidence on Compound 42." Mark Stahmann was not mentioned.

As noted in this narrative, on February 19-20, Stahmann wrote two lengthy letters to the WARF Board of Trustees, detailing what he said were his contributions to the warfarin discovery and patenting. He mentioned having read in the newspapers that "a contract involving this patent is now being negotiated," though warfarin had been selling commercially since the previous summer. Stahmann may have been referring to the patent royalties' contract (in the end, the three inventors split 15 percent). It also seems possible the *Reader's Digest* article – Stahmann could well have seen the March issue by mid-February – prompted his writing to the foundation trustees.

On the last page of his lengthy missive, Stahmann wrote, "I am entitled to public recognition by the Wisconsin Alumni Research Foundation and the University for the part I played in the discovery... of Warfarin."

Stahmann also reached out to Paul de Kruif, wondering why his name was not in the article. De Kruif sent a telegram saying it was in the draft he submitted. "By long distance," de Kruif wrote, "in the presence of Ward Ross, deletion of your and other names was requested by Prof. Link."

9. RATTOR

Reader's Digest editor De Witt Wallace sent Stahmann a letter with an explanation that reflected less poorly on Karl.

"In the original manuscript," Wallace wrote, "Paul de Kruif included your [Stahmann's] name as well as the names of several other people who contributed to the project. Dr. Link felt that if all those persons were named, others should be named too. His solution was to drop them all."

Those were private letters and telegrams. But on March 15, 1951 – while Karl was away in Arizona, visiting his sisters – *The Daily Cardinal* published an unusual scoop.

It was headlined: "'U' Recognizes Three Men in Warfarin Find." The article began:

"The university will recognize three men as the inventors of warfarin – a revolutionary rodenticide developed at the university and expected to earn millions of dollars, informed sources told the Cardinal late last night.

"In the next 'day or so,' the university news service will issue a release correcting the impression that Dr. Karl Paul Link, university biochemist, is the main inventor. It will list as inventors the three scientists on the warfarin patent."

Later, the article noted, "The Cardinal learned that the decision to issue the statement came after Link had received recognition in a national publication for the warfarin work."

Karl was furious, with the university for issuing the release in his absence, with WARF for going along, and – once again – with Harry Steenbock, whom he accused of "being a chief consultant in a design to make me crawl."

Karl's quote was included in a lengthy March 26 *Capital Times* article – a similar story appeared in the *Wisconsin State Journal* – headlined, "Link Says WARF Pressured U. to Issue 'Damaging' Story."

Karl's quotes were from a letter he'd sent the paper. In the letter, Karl denied he'd tried to claim solo credit for warfarin, saying the charge was ridiculous.

"I have publicly given credit to the work of [Ikawa and Stahmann]," he said. "They are listed as inventors with me on the Warfarin patent."

Karl continued, "On two recent public lecture platforms – on Feb. 1, before a Farm and Home Week audience, and on Feb. 8, before Gamma Alpha society – I have charts giving the names of those who have shared in the work. On the second occasion, I specifically gave full credit to the two [other] inventors in my speech."

In the *Wisconsin State Journal*, Karl said the March 15 *Daily Cardinal* story was "designed to damage my reputation as a teacher, scientist and public servant."

There was also, in the *State Journal* story, this irrefutable paragraph: "Link said Sunday that he is the legal project leader of the Warfarin experiment and noted that he is the only person to have full continuity of the various experiments which have grown out of work on sweet clover hay in the past 18 years."

The controversy over credit for the discovery of warfarin faded relatively quickly, and didn't resurface for nearly half a century, when, upon Stahmann's death in 2000, his daughter spoke to a Milwaukee newspaper reporter about her father feeling slighted. In 1951, as noted, any controversy was dwarfed by warfarin's thundering success as a rat poison. Voluminous column inches in newspapers and magazines around the world were devoted to its efficacy.

One such story in the *Wisconsin State Journal* noted how in 1952, Karl would meet in Madison with Dr. Mohan Singh, who worked to protect Marshall Plan food and grain preserves from the scourge of rats. Singh visited with Karl on a United Nations trip to learn how to use warfarin as a rat killer.

Paul de Kruif's article in *Reader's Digest* gave a detailed description of how warfarin worked in an early experiment on a Middleton farm: "The rats didn't seem to know they were eating poison; night after night they came to the sinister bait pots. On the third and fourth nights they came with a slow and measured gait,

9. RATTOR

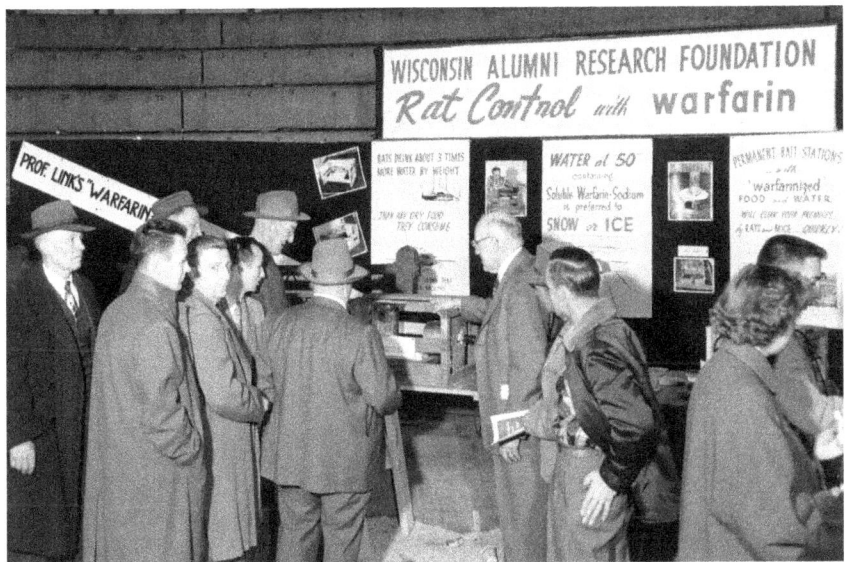

A booth at the UW Stock Pavilion for warfarin, the highly successful rodenticide that subsequently became a widely prescribed human anticoagulant. (UW Archive)

but no bait-shyness. No convulsions. Just painless hemorrhages into their lungs until on the fifth day they were dying, every last rat on that farm dying, peacefully as if going to sleep."

It was perhaps that layer of detail that prompted a postcard from New York City, postmarked March 1951, addressed to "KARL PAUL LINK, KILLER OF DEFENSELESS, VISCONSIN UNIVERSITY, VISCONSIN."

Despite the vague address and the misspelling of Wisconsin, the card made it to Karl, who saved it. The card, not entirely coherent, read in part:

"Karl Paul Link, of Visconsin University

"Your mind thinks only of your own benefit, and those you make on the poor defenseless animals creatures for so much killing YOU MAKE ON THIS EARTH ON NATURE CREATURES YOU WILL SO MUCH ETERNALLY BE TORTURED IN A HELL OF AGONY.... YOU SHALL DIE AGAIN AND AGAIN IN THE SAME HORRIBLE TORTURE WHICH YOU

INFLICT ON DEFENSELESS LITTLE CREATURES. IF RATS WERE GIVEN A CHANCE TO LIVE ON EARTH LIKE OTHER CREATURES THERE WILL BE LESS CORRUPTION... LESS WAR ON EARTH AND NO DESTRUCTION SOON OF ALL THE EARTH BY ATOM BOMB."

The card was not signed. Karl, who proudly claimed the label "Rattor" for the rest of his life, may have found some irony in his correspondent's atomic bomb reference. Karl spoke often – publicly – of the terrible dangers of atomic proliferation. But he had no qualms about killing rats. Moreover, Karl would soon see yet another highly consequential application for warfarin, this time in a way to medically benefit humans. It would lead to a series of prestigious international awards and carry Karl to the very pinnacle of his profession.

Not untypically, before that could happen, there was one more controversy.

10. CALF SCOURS AND UNPOPULAR CAUSES

KARL'S INTEREST IN CALF SCOURS – the source of a clash that would eventually lead to his censure by the UW Board of Regents – dated back more than a decade, to 1938.

He and the students in his lab were closing in on isolating what in spoiled sweet clover was causing the blood of cows to not coagulate. Their tests involved laboratory animals, including rabbits, but Karl and his team were frustrated by the number of newborn rabbits that didn't live long enough to become test subjects.

"Out of every litter of new rabbits," Karl said later, "a third would die, at best. At worst, they might all die."

Karl recalled an article he had read on scours, which is not a single disease but rather a clinical diagnosis of numerous illnesses marked by severe diarrhea. Newborns die from dehydration. One antidote for young calves – which are particularly vulnerable – involved antibodies present in the heavy milk, called colostrum, of a mother cow immediately after birth. Working with cow blood, Karl was able to develop a serum "which contained the antibodies," according to a later *State Journal* article.

"He mixed Vitamin K with the blood serum," the *State Journal* noted, "so that the two would work simultaneously, and he fed it to his rabbits, and it worked!" A large percentage of the baby rabbits survived. The vitamin helped forestall any hemorrhaging.

Would it work on animals beyond rabbits? Karl thought it might, and it could prove important, because for whatever reason

– perhaps something to do with modern farming techniques – calves were less often receiving the necessary colostrum from their mothers' milk.

Of course, Karl soon became preoccupied with the pursuit of the anticoagulant dicumarol. Calf scours were not top of mind. Years passed. Karl would later say that in that interim University of Wisconsin administrators and academics in departments other than his own prevented his access to the cows and calves with which he might have been able to advance his scours research.

Finally, in the late 1940s, and with encouragement from the pharmaceutical company E. R. Squibb and Sons – Ward Ross from WARF brought Karl together with them – Karl struck a deal to take his work on calf scours off the UW campus to Asheville, North Carolina, where a herd of some 1,400 cows lived on the famed Biltmore property.

In March 1952, *The Country Gentleman*, a national agriculture magazine with more than a century's history, published an enthusiastic story about Karl's work in North Carolina.

"A new preventative treatment for calf scours," the piece noted, "promises to lick the virulent septicemia which frequently kills young calves in their first few days of life."

The *Country Gentleman* article came out in late March 1952, and reporters from the *Wisconsin State Journal* and *The Capital Times* quickly asked Karl why a scientist of his stature had found himself taking his research out of Wisconsin.

Karl's answers begat another campus controversy, more headlines, and finally a censure.

It should be noted that just a week earlier, Karl received notice that he'd won a prestigious award, the Cameron Prize, from the University of Edinburgh in Scotland. The letter from the university's medical faculty explained:

"The Cameron Prize, of the value of about 150 Pounds Sterling, is awarded annually to 'a person who, in the course of the five years immediately preceding, has made any highly important and valuable addition to practical therapeutics.' In your

10. CALF SCOURS AND UNPOPULAR CAUSES

case it is awarded in recognition of your work on anti-coagulant therapy as exemplified by the introduction of dicumarol, which was entirely the result of investigation undertaken in your laboratory and under your direction.

"Its discovery has opened up a wide field of therapeutics, with practical reference to the prevention and treatment of thrombotic phenomena."

Karl was especially pleased to receive the prize from the University of Edinburgh, located just 40 miles south of St. Andrews, where he studied in the 1920s. Indeed, an Edinburgh professor who had also been at St. Andrews sent Karl a congratulatory note:

"Our medical faculty is truly Scotch with the Cameron award. It is given only for contributions that will stick in medical practice. The 1951 award went jointly to T. Reichstein and E. C. Kendal for their work on cortisone. I salute you, fellow St. Andrian, on this recognition."

Reichstein and Kendal shared the Nobel Prize in 1950.

On March 23, Karl sent a letter to Sydney Smith, Dean of the Faculty of Medicine at Edinburgh, accepting the award. Smith wrote back inviting Karl to receive the prize in person and give a lecture on dicumarol in July.

Karl didn't make it to Scotland, at least not then.

As John Newhouse wrote in the *Wisconsin State Journal*, six years later, in 1958: "Dr. Link still has the money in the bank for a trip to the University of Edinburgh, in Scotland. Back in 1952, he was awarded the highly regarded Cameron Prize… and asked to Scotland to make a speech and receive the award. The only trouble was that he was engaged in one of his classic brawls. So he sent the dean of Edinburgh a letter which said, in effect, that he was engaged in an interesting fight and that – if they'd put the travel expenses in the bank – he'd come over later on. They did."

(Karl made it not to Scotland but England in the early 1970s, when he and his wife, Elizabeth, traveled to Cambridge University for a dinner honoring the great protein chemist A. C. Chibnall. It was at the dinner that Karl asked Chibnall's wife – a Latin scholar – for the Latin translation of the phrase he wanted for his epitaph: "He gave rats an easy out.")

The brawl – to use reporter Newhouse's term – that kept Karl stateside in 1952 concerned his calf scours research. Reached by *The Capital Times* after *The Country Gentleman* article appeared, Karl said he and WARF made "an attempt to get the testing done in Wisconsin, but that fizzled." Karl said he'd received written permission from Dr. Conrad Elvehjem, dean of the graduate school and chairman of the university research committee, to take his research to North Carolina. Elvehjem denied granting written permission, saying it was unnecessary, telling the *State Journal* that professors "are free to do as they please in matters such as these."

Karl was incensed – or acted so. "Defection!" he told the *State Journal*. "I didn't think Elvehjem would do it! My mind is now made up. I shall write a letter to Frank J. Sensenbrenner asking an investigation before the Board of Regents." (Sensenbrenner, of Neenah, was the board president.)

That story appeared March 26.

The next day, Karl stepped up his attack.

A prominent March 27 *State Journal* headline read: "Link Says Fred, Baldwin 'Blocked' Test Work Here."

The story, by John Newhouse, began: "Dr. Karl Paul Link, University of Wisconsin biochemist, Wednesday night charged that Pres. E. B. Fred and Vice-President Ira L. Baldwin of the university were the two top administrators who blocked him in his attempt to have work on calf scours performed at the university."

Baldwin could not be reached for comment; Fred claimed not to remember: "I'd have to look it up in my files."

Newhouse reported that Karl also sent a letter to Sensenbrenner, asking for a formal investigation.

On March 28, Fred, the UW president issued a statement: "Throughout the years, Dr. Link and his work have had generous support. During this period, it has been impossible to give our

10. CALF SCOURS AND UNPOPULAR CAUSES

research workers all of the aid and facilities which their work would seem to justify... Dr. Link has had, in line with the Wisconsin tradition, the usual freedom in planning and carrying on his own research and teaching. In spite of limitation of facilities, Dr. Link has been very productive and has made some outstanding discoveries. We hope his investigations related to calf scours will prove of great value."

Karl called Fred's statement "very fine buck passing."

On April 10, Karl got his wish: He was invited to appear before the Board of Regents. The meeting was held in Bascom Hall. Elvehjem, Fred, and Baldwin were in attendance, along with Karl and the regents. Karl joined the group at 4:20 p.m. and was introduced to Helen Laird, a new regent and mother of future congressman and secretary of defense Melvin Laird. Karl next went around shaking hands with the other regents, then took his seat.

Sensenbrenner began, "Mr. Link is here in respect to a request received from him under the date of March 26 to appear before the Regents. I would like to ask him to get down to business. I will ask him a direct question; perhaps he can answer 'yes' or 'no' to that question." Sensenbrenner then asked Karl if he had any complaint against the university administration regarding its treatment of him in areas like projects assigned or facilities furnished.

Sensenbrenner might have hoped for a yes or no answer, but what he got was a five-minute soliloquy.

"That's a loaded question," Karl began, and then related his unsuccessful on and off efforts during the decade of the 1940s to get animals for testing for his calf scours research – the inaction that drove him to North Carolina.

Helen Laird, noting that was in the past, asked Karl, "What is your gripe now?"

Before Karl could answer, Sensenbrenner added – and this would prove to be the central concern of the regents – "Why the shooting in the newspapers?"

Karl's answer: "Toward the end of one of the articles I said, 'There is nothing to gain for me, but something to be gained for the campus.' There are young men on the campus better than I am who cannot get through on problems where situations are comparable to what we have now."

The meeting wore on, and it became apparent that for the most part no one really disputed Karl's version of events – other than Elvehjem insisting he hadn't given Karl written permission to take his work off campus – but what upset the administration and the regents was Karl's being critical of them in the press.

Regent Sensenbrenner: "Where did [John Newhouse of the *State Journal*] get the information in the first place?"

Karl: "From this article in *The Country Gentleman*. Does a reporter have the right to ask 'why?' I think he does."

(Newhouse had called Karl after seeing the magazine piece and said, "Why in the devil did you go to North Carolina? Isn't this the Dairy State?" Karl replied, "John, if I answer that I'm on the spot," then proceeded to answer it.)

Regent Wilbur Renk: "You have stated certain accusations against the president and Vice President Baldwin in the newspapers and blew the university up."

Karl: "I think the university can survive more than this."

Regent W. J. Campbell: "It was sensational."

Karl: "You think I bought that space?"

Regent Campbell: "Did the reporters come to you when they wrote that article?"

Karl: "Certainly they came to me... I'll tell you, gentlemen, I did not buy that space."

Two months later, in June 1952, the Board of Regents voted to censure Karl. A report from the board's personnel committee read in part:

"It is the opinion of the Regents that the charges made by Dr. Link were without any foundation whatsoever. The making of such unwarranted accusations is unfair to the individuals concerned and detrimental to the University; and Dr. Link is subject to censure for having broadcast such unwarranted charges."

10. CALF SCOURS AND UNPOPULAR CAUSES

Note that Karl's basic "charge" – that his attempts to do the work on campus were not encouraged – was not specifically refuted. The suspicion remains that the real problem was Karl talking to the press. In any case he issued his own statement: "The big question remains – why was the university not interested? I do not know the answer and apparently the Regent committee didn't take the time to find out… The Regents should be more than a rubber stamp to the administrators of the university. I grieved for the state of Wisconsin this afternoon. I saw that stamp in action."

Years later, Karl would make much of the fact that in the same meeting in which he was censured, he was also voted a $500 raise in annual salary (to $11,360).

Karl's demeanor in meetings – be it with faculty colleagues or the Board of Regents – usually contained more than a bit of theater. Henry Lardy, who was on the faculty of the Enzyme Institute, described it this way in an Oral History Program interview:

"Whenever the faculty met and Karl chose to come, which wasn't very often, he brought with him, under one arm, a large can of Edgeworth tobacco. It looked like about a three-pound coffee can. [Also] His dinner pail, which had in it a bottle of beer and a thermos of coffee. There was a long ritual involved immediately after his arrival. The dinner pail would be opened, the coffee would be poured, he'd fill his pipe – which took many matches to get lit – and this was going on while deliberations of great importance to the department were being discussed."

Lardy concluded, "I think it was mainly for show because he was flamboyant in every conceivable way. He usually did not participate in discussions. Sometimes, but usually he was silent."

Lardy, it should be noted, was fond of Karl. In the same interview, he noted, "I enjoyed visiting with [Karl] a great deal because I was interested in carbohydrates and a lot of the work being done in his laboratory… He was marvelously cooperative to anyone who was civil to him. He was a splendid person, really a marvelous person."

Karl's calf scours skirmish with the Board of Regents – and regents Sensenbrenner and Campbell in particular – was well documented in the press. Less well documented – but hugely important in locating the intellectual integrity at the core of Karl's character – was an earlier clash with Sensenbrenner and Campbell that was ignited by Karl's support of leftist student organizations on the UW campus.

In his National Academies biograph of Karl, Robert Burris inexplicably denigrates the seriousness of Karl's commitment to certain political ideas and organizations.

"People tend to play up Link as a great liberal and defender of unpopular causes," Burris wrote. "For example, some biographical records praise him as being against Joe McCarthy. On the UW campus during the McCarthy era, one was hard pressed to find anyone on the faculty who was for McCarthy. Link did serve as faculty sponsor for certain left-wing groups (the John Cookson Karl Marx Discussion Group, the Labor Youth League…) In my opinion, Link did not really embrace and actively promote any radical causes, but he was happy to serve as front man."

An examination of Karl's support of the two campus groups named by Burris completely contradicts Burris's conclusion.

Included in Karl's archive at UW is a lengthy report he delivered to UW President E.B. Fred in 1957 about his involvement with both the Cookson Marxist Discussion Group and the Youth Labor League (Karl also gave a speech on the subject to the Madison Literary Club on the night of the day he gave his report to Fred – January 14, 1957).

In his report to Fred, Karl noted that it was with some hesitation that he agreed to serve as faculty adviser to the John Cookson Marxist Discussion Club (in 1947) and (in 1950, after that club ceased operation) the Labor Youth League.

"Originally I was reluctant to serve," Karl noted.

10. CALF SCOURS AND UNPOPULAR CAUSES

His reasoning was that the clubs might be better served by a historian or political scientist than a biochemist. Yet in each case the clubs could not find a faculty member willing to sign on as adviser, and without one, they would lack official standing on campus (which happened to those groups at other universities).

Given that situation, Karl agreed to serve as adviser, noting he had "a sound base for accepting the faculty advisership to unpopular student organizations."

It went back, Karl noted, to things learned in the Link home when he was growing up in Indiana.

"We were taught that the Declaration of Independence and the Bill of Rights were among the greatest political instruments ever forged in Western Civilization," Karl wrote. "People of all faiths, of all parties, of all economic levels, of all trades and professions frequented our house. Anyone holding a different political view from the one traditional in our household was not regarded as a suspicious or traitorous character. However, my father was hard on cheats, liars and cowards. Matters of the spirit had value – conscience was recognized – and in the courtroom he frequently showed his preference for justice over law.

"We were taught principles and to stick to them," Karl continued. "We were also taught not to accept any verbal, written or physical bullying. Cognizance of the risks of being unpopular – alone on issues – was in the warp and woof of my training before I came here as a freshman in September 1918.

"It is from these teachings and experiences at home that I accepted the faculty advisership to the LYL and its predecessor. I offer no apology for my predilections. As a result of my having accepted the advisership to LYL etc., I have been labelled, in private and in public, 'parlor-pinko, dupe, fellow traveler, campus-commie, un-American, egg-head, long-haired subversive' – these and more have come my way."

In late 1946 and early 1947, before the Cookson Marxist group was officially recognized at UW-Madison, Karl said he was contacted by Regent F. J. Sensenbrenner, "who indicated in no uncertain terms that if I accepted the advisership the consequences for me would be serious."

At the same time, another regent, W.J. Campbell, contacted Karl, and, in attempting to dissuade him, Karl said, voiced "his intention to counteract 'subversive student clubs' through a required course in American history for all students."

Karl's response to Campbell?

"I told him repeatedly," Karl wrote, "that English, Arithmetic, Biology, Chemistry and the History of Western Political Philosophies were just as important as the Boston Tea Party and/or the amount of whisky consumed by the brilliant General Grant, and that his efforts would be better spent if he made an attempt to raise the general level of high school teaching in Wisconsin."

Karl noted that despite their sharp political differences, his conversations with Campbell were not antagonistic.

"Mr. Campbell was always polite," Karl wrote. "Always decent. He always tried to persuade me and we consistently parted on friendly terms."

On one occasion, Campbell proffered a compromise. He would not object to a Labor Youth League chapter in Madison if the faculty adviser provided the Regents and/or the administration a membership list.

Karl was not impressed. "I indicated that if the adviser had to be an informer, I would not serve."

Contrasting Campbell with Sensenbrenner, his other Regent critic, Karl noted that Sensenbrenner's "approach was that of a firm believer in self-constituted authority."

By the end of 1952, Karl's problems with the Board of Regents regarding the leftist student groups eased – Campbell cycled off the board and Sensenbrenner died.

"(They) were the only members of the Board who tried to throttle me," Karl wrote, "and after the death of Sensenbrenner my contacts with the Regents on the LYL issue ceased."

Karl's last meeting with Sensenbrenner, the president and chairman of the board of Kimberly-Clark, was memorable.

10. CALF SCOURS AND UNPOPULAR CAUSES

According to Karl, he was summoned to Sensenbrenner's hospital bedside at Wisconsin General in Madison.

Karl recalled that Sensenbrenner said, "I have never seen the likes of you!" He accused Karl of causing him trouble and costing the university money. Karl noted that Sensenbrenner said "he had the authority to displace me."

Sensenbrenner's final salvo was this: "When LYL and the other campus subversives are investigated by Washington, you will be the first to go along with those Reds!"

In his report to UW President Fred, Karl recalled his reaction to that statement: "I managed to remain as composed as a submerged rock in a Norwegian fjord."

Karl, in his report, then thanked President Fred and the balance of the Board of Regents for not buckling to the threats of Campbell and Sensenbrenner. Karl quoted Princeton Professor H. H. Wilson, who wrote in 1952: "Too few of us seem aware of the relationship between freedom of speech or association… and the survival of democratic politics."

Karl included in the report what transpired when he went to hear two speakers invited to campus by the Labor Youth League.

The first, in January 1953, was Abner Berry, the African American editor of the Harlem edition of the *Daily Worker* newspaper.

"Some local vigilantes had called on me the afternoon of the meeting," Karl noted. They threatened reprisal if Berry spoke as scheduled.

"In a potential dog-eat-dog fiesta and/or political climate," Karl recalled, "I had no intention of being clawed, bitten or eaten. So I hired a seasoned guard (unarmed of course) to go with me. I do not relate this with glee in my heart, but when someone comes to tell you that, 'You and your ilk are not wanted, and we will do so and so if the meeting is held,' one either folds or one takes appropriate protective steps."

That night, Karl noted, "Fortunately nothing overt transpired. I saw two of the four threateners at the meeting – spoke to them – congratulated them on their behavior and shook hands before I left about 10:45 p.m."

A little less than two years later, Karl intercepted three students as they entered the Memorial Union where Leon Wofsy was about to address a campus audience in Tripp Commons. Wofsy was a Labor Youth League leader, and, later, a distinguished scientist and free speech advocate at the University of California-Berkeley. He was also Jewish.

The three students Karl stopped held a large placard that they intended to place at the Tripp Commons entrance. The sign read: "KIKES."

"I was able to convince them," Karl noted, "that their stunt would be an actionable act and managed to acquire the board without difficulty."

There were other incidents, including a Pete Seeger concert promoted by the LYL – under Karl's signature – that drew Young Republican picketers, but no violence.

The LYL folded on the Madison campus in fall 1956. Karl's report to President Fred (and his speech on the subject to the Madison Literary Club) came a few months later.

Toward the end of his report, Karl summarized his feelings about the decade he spent advising the politically unpopular student groups. He felt history would vindicate him.

"Prediction in any field of human activity is hazardous," Karl wrote, "but I am quite confident that when the historians assemble the facts and weigh them objectively with benefit of 'time's clear perspective' they will write that the faculty adviser to LYL and the like during the years 1946-57 came home – somewhat battered, to be sure, by his methods – but he still had the shield of honest thought."

Karl's stirring conclusion: "I hasten to tell you that I do not look upon this work as a divine mission divinely performed. No, I see myself quite clearly as a campus trouper – whose pants were already frayed at the cuffs when I took the job in 1947. A job had to be done and it was my good fortune to be in a position to do it…

10. Calf Scours and Unpopular Causes

"I now close by restating the last two paragraphs from the letter that I wrote to the Student Life and Interest Committee in February 1953:

"'I firmly believe in helping to keep alive the American spirit of free inquiry on our campus. This is perhaps the greatest service that I have rendered the University in twenty-six (now thirty) years that I have served on its faculty. I find it appropriate to close with the words of Abraham Lincoln: When you begin qualifying freedom watch out for the consequences to you.'"

In June 1955, a year before the LYL folded, Karl and Elizabeth's oldest son, John Kailin Link, graduated from Wisconsin High School, located on the UW-Madison campus. A vote of the graduating seniors brought an invitation for Karl to make the commencement address. Some time earlier, the Republican U.S. senator from Wisconsin, Alexander Wiley, had addressed the students and apparently not impressed them. After Wiley's speech, one of the seniors got word to Karl: "Don't give us the usual feed."

He did not. Karl's commencement address – eventually reprinted in *The Capital Times* – was a passionate defense of the record of the late U. S. President Franklin D. Roosevelt and a warning about the dangers of xenophobia and the diatribes of another U.S. senator from Wisconsin, Joseph McCarthy.

Speaking to the students of FDR, Karl said, "When most of you were eight years old, he died suddenly from a brain hemorrhage. You have only a fringe memory of the sorrow and concern that his death caused."

Karl noted: "The period of 1933-45 while Roosevelt was president has been referred to by Wisconsin's junior senator [McCarthy] as 'the period of treason.'"

Karl scoffed and noted, "It was 'treason' to set up legislative machinery to put the American economic system back into operation in 1933 when a severe depression gripped and nearly strangled this country. 'Treason' to assemble the best talent available – regardless of party affiliation – for the problems at hand.

"It was 'treason' to feed hungry people when agricultural surpluses were going to waste on our farms. 'Treason' to protect our soil, to rehabilitate river valleys via TVA and the like to bring electricity into the rural areas. It was 'treason' to put the jobless to work. 'Treason' to provide decent housing, to help writers, artists, poets, playwrights, scholars, actors and scientists, professional people of all kinds, through government sponsored work projects. It was 'treason' to aid countries fighting Hitler and Mussolini. And here is the nub. It was 'treason' to go into war against Hitler and Mussolini."

Concluding, Karl urged the students to read Milton Crane's book, "The Roosevelt Era," adding, "You can gain hope, courage and wisdom by understanding America's record during the first ten years of your life. And so as you come of age, work diligently to develop your talents. Work is the best thing to make us love life. But carry yourselves beyond school and work by reading widely. Study and weigh that which may not be approved by the McCarthyites. Oppose any form of tyranny over the mind of men. Without freedom of thought and expression no man is free."

The publication of the address in *The Capital Times* brought at least a couple of vitriolic responses.

One was from a man named Frank Harris, who owned a lumber company in Boaz, in Richland County, and on whose stationery was stamped: "Because all communists, reds and radicals hate Joe McCarthy, I am for him."

Harris wrote a letter to the *Wisconsin State Journal* and copied Karl.

"[Karl] evidently assumes this would be the last brain-washing these kids would get, so he really made it good… glorifying the Roosevelts…the usual sneering remarks concerning our most courageous Senator McCarthy…. The walls of our indignation overflow when we witness our children being brain-washed with this propaganda."

A man named Verne Kaub, evidently an inveterate writer of letters to newspapers, wrote *The Capital Times* with this: "The

10. CALF SCOURS AND UNPOPULAR CAUSES

balance of the address was a defense of all the worst features of the Roosevelt regime, scoffing at all those who are brave enough to designate monstrous 'mistakes' of Roosevelt as what they really are, which is treason."

In an editorial printed the same time, *The Capital Times* editorial board addressed Kaub's letter, saying this: "Kaub shows that he has been picked up and swept along on the wave of hysteria, which McCarthy and his clique promoted and exploited. For a man to charge a former president, four times elected by the people, with treason indicates how deeply the now waning torrents of hysteria have been running in this country."

11. WARFARIN FOR PEOPLE

PERHAPS DUE TO HIS REPEATED jousting with regents Campbell and Sensenbrenner in the late '40s and early '50s, Karl's ambivalence toward the UW Board of Regents never abated. In 1973, he was profiled in *The Daily Cardinal* student newspaper, and the regents came up.

"What do they know about education?" Karl asked. "They're nothing but a bunch of businessmen."

As time went on, Karl's antipathy toward "the establishment" would figure into most of the many profiles written about him, and indeed be included in eulogies after his death.

One of the latter came from an academic colleague, Einar Haugen, who noted, "He loved to tease his friends, but he could be merciless in his criticism of dishonesty and cowardice in his colleagues or university officials."

From a UW news release upon Karl's 1971 retirement: "He has never hesitated to stand up for his beliefs, even if they caused trouble for him. Prof. Link often has disagreed with colleagues, administrators and politicians."

Clay Schoenfeld, in an unpublished history of WARF, put it this way: "For a generation Link made campus life more relevant than it might otherwise have been, certainly more interesting if not downright exciting. Flamboyant and mercurial like his fellow Badger, Frank Lloyd Wright, staunch devotee of the Bill of Rights, Link seemed to take a positive delight in tweaking the tails of any defenders of the status quo, to the end that he became a hero to humanities students of the radical fringe and the bête noire of conservative Trustees and Regents."

11. Warfarin for People

The most benign description of Karl's confrontations with authority came from the journalist John Newhouse – who knew Karl well – and may deserve to be the most enduring:

"It isn't quite right, however, to call these encounters brawls," Newhouse wrote. "Dr. Link embarks on them in high good humor, cherishes his opponents, and winds up on friendly terms with them."

Well, most of them, anyway.

Somewhat ironically, for all the angst and handwringing over the calf scours research – it was eventually patented as Plasmylac – it didn't produce the desired long-term results. As Don Behm put it in his biographical memoir of Karl: "Several years later, a 'fool proof' serum still evaded Karl and his colleagues from the Department of Genetics."

The same would not be said of the evolution across the decade of the 1950s of another of Karl's discoveries.

It began in a most unlikely way, as described in the opening paragraph of an article years later in *Distillations*, the magazine of the Science History Institute:

"On April 4, 1951, a 22-year-old military inductee stumbled into a naval hospital in Philadelphia. Doubled over with acute back and abdominal pain, he could barely walk. As nurses tried to secure him to a gurney, his nose began to bleed profusely; a flood of red spilled over his clothes. After several hours doctors managed to stabilize him, but they couldn't figure out what had caused the bleeding. Some suspected he had been poisoned. But with what? And by whom?"

In his famous 1958 New York City lecture on the discovery of dicumarol and warfarin, Karl picked up the story: "On April 5, we were informed by Captain J. Love (MC) in the U.S.N. at Philadelphia that an army inductee was admitted to the Naval Hospital who had taken over a period of five days a concentrate of warfarin designed for rodent control."

In his inimitable way, Karl noted that while "the inductee had followed the multiple dose directions on the package, it became clear to him that w0arfarin was not an efficient agent to shuffle off this mortal coil." Karl took those last words from Hamlet's famous "To Be or Not to Be" speech in Shakespeare.

The *Distillations* article noted, "The recruit was despondent as he told his tale, but his doctors were intrigued."

The doctors would eventually publish accounts of his case in medical journals in 1952 and 1953. In the meantime, in Madison, Karl viewed the story out of Philadelphia as "a catalyst." Maybe warfarin – or, more precisely, the water-soluble sodium salt of warfarin (warfarin sodium) – could be a safe yet more effective anticoagulant in humans than dicumarol. Karl had one of his students, Collin Schroeder, working to perfect the process of making warfarin sodium.

In January 1953, Karl was in touch with two friendly physician investigators, Shepard Shapiro in New York and Ovid Meyer in Madison, about commencing clinical trials. He had also interested a longtime friend, Dr. Samuel Gordon, vice president of the pharmaceutical company Endo Products, in manufacturing the drug.

Gordon had originally been fearful that the name warfarin – so prevalent as a rat poison – might give pause to humans considering it as a medicine.

But in a January 28, 1953 letter to Karl, Gordon wrote that "I have overcome my fears regarding the name warfarin and Warfarin Sodium. I have no fear now that Warfarin (or its sodium derivative) need be referred to in medicine as a rat poison."

In early letters to clinicians, Gordon referred to the drug as Compound 42, then Coumadin Sodium, the name under which it would eventually be marketed. But it was warfarin, all right, and it worked in humans. Indeed, it worked wonders.

The *Distillations* article summed it up nicely:

"Early trials revealed that Warfarin could do everything dicumarol could but with several times the potency. When an arterial blood clot in or near the brain caused a stroke, Warfarin was able to restore the blood flow and prevent another stroke.

11. Warfarin for People

And when patients lay in bed for long periods after surgery, Warfarin prevented the slow-moving blood in their leg veins from clotting. Whereas dicumarol's effects were often delayed and short lived, Warfarin had immediate and long-lasting effects, regardless of whether it was delivered orally or intravenously. Paradoxically, the properties that differentiated Warfarin from dicumarol made it both a better rat poison and better medicine in humans."

In 1953, it was still the rat poison that was making news. On March 3, a former student of Karl's, Dorothy Wu, who had helped in the lab perfecting warfarin in the late 1940s when it was still known as Compound 42, wrote Karl a letter from California. Wu and another student of Karl's, Clint Ballou, had married and were living in Berkeley.

Wu began by congratulating Karl on an article on warfarin as rat killer in a recent issue of *The Farm Quarterly*, joking that the writer had compared Karl's appearance to a "western movie star" with "dark floating hair and a stern profile."

Wu's reason for writing, she said, was that a press officer from the U.S. State Department was in touch with her about a proposed article on Wu's contribution to the warfarin discovery. Two different Far East magazines – one in Manila, the other in Hong Kong – were interested. Wu wanted Karl's opinion on whether she should cooperate. Karl not only enthusiastically endorsed the stories, he contacted John Newhouse at the *Wisconsin State Journal* asking Newhouse to send Wu copies of the photos he had of her in Karl's lab – another small example of Karl going to bat for his students.

On March 5, 1953, two days after Wu wrote to Karl, an event of surpassing importance worldwide occurred – Soviet dictator Joseph Stalin died. But it would be 50 years before anyone suggested the role warfarin may have played in the death.

Such speculation is at odds with the idea that warfarin couldn't cause a human to "shuffle off this mortal coil," as Karl phrased it. Yet in sufficient quantity, perhaps it could, and did, in the case of Stalin, whose generals were known to fear he was becoming increasingly unhinged.

The poisoning theory was advanced in a 2003 book, "Stalin's Last Crime," written by Yale professor Joseph Brent and Russian historian Vladimir Naumov.

The author of this narrative interviewed Brent at the time of the book's publication. We spoke by phone on March 5, 2003 – 50 years to the day after Stalin died.

I wrote a newspaper column about the book and the theory. A warm and humorous letter arrived a few days later, written by Frederick Bauch of Carefree, Arizona, Bauch explained that while a student at UW-Madison in the 1940s, he got a job as a "mail clerk and gofer" at WARF. Bauch continued: "One of my jobs was to buy a case of Budweiser in cans and put it in the refrigerator in the Biochem lab for Dr. Karl Paul Link every Friday afternoon. While I was helping him, he invented warfarin. [Many] years later, in 1997, I developed a blood clot in my leg. The Coumadin [the trade name for warfarin] they gave me dissolved the clot before it reached my lung and saved my life. I helped Dr. Link and he saved my life."

The "Stalin's Last Crime" authors had unearthed the official medical account of Stalin's demise given to the Communist Party Central Committee three months after his death. A cerebral hemorrhage was the widely circulated cause of death, but the documents revealed there had also been severe stomach bleeding. Might the worried generals have poisoned him?

Brent gave the medical records to two doctors he knew at Yale.

"They both said the same thing," Brent told me. "They said the cause of death was either cerebral hemorrhage or warfarin poisoning."

Brent had never heard of warfarin, but he did some research and wound up on the phone with Howard Bremer, WARF's long-time patent attorney in Madison.

11. WARFARIN FOR PEOPLE

"We get a lot of funny calls," Bremer said, sometime later. "But this one was interesting."

In the end, no definitive conclusion was reached on what killed Stalin. Speculation remains irresistible.

"Wouldn't it be interesting," Brent said, "if one of the biggest rats in history was killed by rat poison?"

Back in 1953, of course, no one at WARF, nor Karl, would have wanted to hear that. They were busy preparing to present warfarin sodium to the world as a superior human anticoagulant.

Meanwhile, in June 1953, Karl and Elizabeth welcomed their third and final son, Paul, to the world.

Among the many congratulatory notes was a letter from Mary Niemann, wife of Carl Niemann, one of Karl's earliest students in his lab in Madison. Niemann became a highly distinguished faculty member at Caltech in Pasadena and was elected to the National Academy of Sciences in 1952.

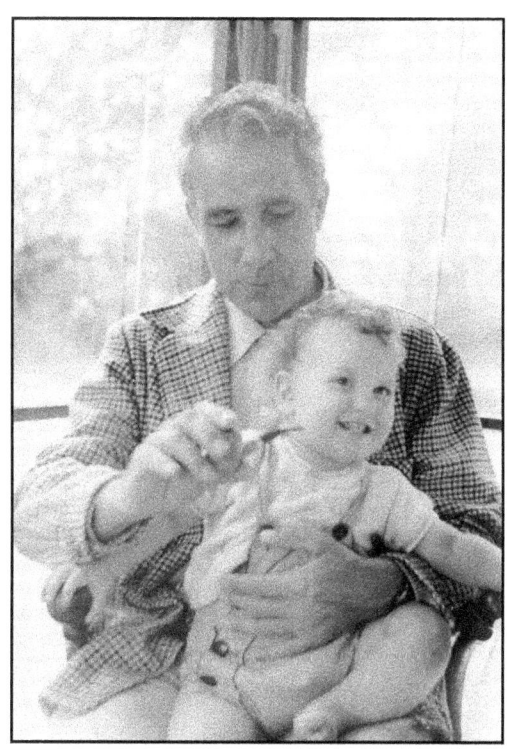

Karl and his youngest son, Paul. (Link family)

"A pitcher, a catcher and third baseman," Mary Niemann wrote, referencing the three Link boys. "Are you going to stop short of a shortstop? All kidding aside, we rejoice in your happiness and wish Paul Konrad Karl Link a long and happy life."

The close connection between Karl – and Elizabeth – and his students can also be seen in a Feb. 4, 1955 note from Bill Stone, a recent student embarking on a career in genetics. Elizabeth had hosted a party at the Highlands home to celebrate Karl's 54th birthday on Jan. 31, and Stone's note was to her.

"I would be doing a great injustice," Stone wrote, "were I not to thank you again for a most delightful evening in celebration of Dr. Link's birthday. I hope that I was not rude in leaving earlier than the other fellows, but my day of bleeding cows etc. began at 6:30 a.m. the next morning. Armed with the lingering smells and tastes of the fabulous food and drinks of the previous evening my day was indeed a pleasant one. Thank you again."

By late 1953, clinicians around the country were beginning trials with warfarin sodium, testing its efficacy as a human anticoagulant. Numerous heart physicians received letters like this one sent by Karl's friend and colleague Samuel Gordon, vice president of Eno Products, in June 1953 to Dr. Joseph Spitzer, a heart specialist at the New York University Cardiac Clinic.

"Dear Dr. Spitzer," Gordon wrote, "Dr. Karl Paul Link of the University of Wisconsin has made available to us a small supply of his Coumadin Sodium (Warfarin-sodium derivative), from which we prepared an injection solution for use as an [anti-clotting] agent.... Will you not complete the investigator's form and return it? As you are aware, we regard Coumadin Sodium as a new drug within the terms of the Food, Drug and Cosmetic Act."

Two years on – in May 1955 – Gordon wrote Karl an enthusiastic letter about the drug's reception, noting that while it is great when friendly physicians like Shapiro and Meyer responded favorably, "it is quite another when we begin to hear it

11. Warfarin for People

from the sticks. The true value of a drug for which a large segment of our population are potential candidates must of necessity come from the sticks… That is coming slowly but surely…"

Gordon shared five recent responses with Karl, all similar to this note from a surgeon in Syracuse: "In general, we have been very well impressed with this new anticoagulant. We have been joined in our enthusiasm by other surgeons in Syracuse, who have used a part of our complimentary supply."

Gordon concluded, "More such letters appear to be coming. A few don't make a lake, but they do indicate a trend. Physicians as a rule are chary with good words for a drug product."

Near the end of his 1958 New York Academy of Medicine speech, Karl would summarize the early, positive warfarin/Coumadin results in human patients:

"Today it would appear… that most of the drawbacks of dicumarol have been overcome. Warfarin sodium is at least five and possibly ten times more potent than dicumarol. It is the only synthetic anticoagulant available today for therapeutic anticoagulation that can be given orally, intravenously, intramuscularly, or rectally. The rate of absorption is almost the same, irrespective of how it is administered. No other anticoagulant of the dicumarol type has all these virtues. Of course, an overdosage can be readily corrected via vitamin K… It is my firm belief it will replace dicumarol on the basis of its performance over a wide variety of conditions and that other anticoagulants of the dicumarol type will not be superior."

In late summer 1955, just as the early returns from Coumadin were coming in, Karl received word that he would be receiving the Albert Lasker Award from the American Public Health Association. The Lasker Awards, launched a decade earlier, reward individuals and groups for outstanding contributions in research related to death and disability-causing diseases. They quickly became one of the most prestigious awards in medicine, often a precursor to an individual winning the Nobel Prize.

The Lasker Awards ceremony was scheduled for October in Kansas City, Missouri. Karl's award was for medical research and the program citation included this: "In view of the vast numbers of individuals affected by thromboembolic diseases each year and the fundamental steps taken by Dr. Link toward the solution of these problems, he has earned the deep gratitude of the medical profession and the lay public of this and coming generations."

Former United States President Harry Truman gave the keynote address at the ceremony and in it congratulated the association on honoring "a University of Wisconsin biochemist who has given us a new weapon against coronary thrombosis."

Also that fall of 1955, a note – sent to the University of Wisconsin News Service – arrived saying that *Life* magazine was interested in possibly profiling Karl. Would it be possible for Karl

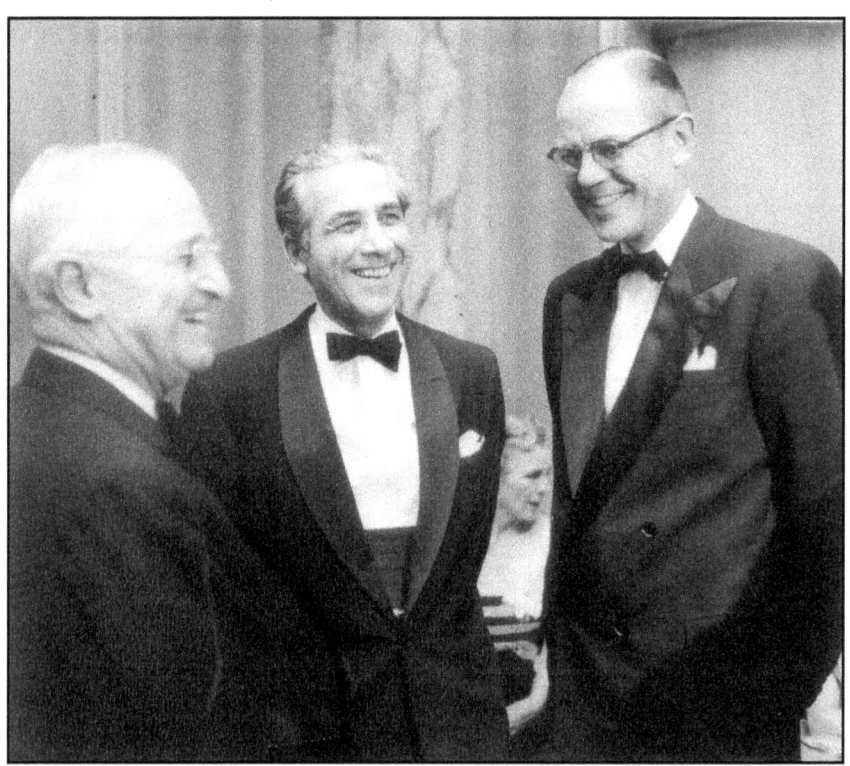

Former President Harry Truman, Karl Paul Link, and Gaylord W. Anderson at the 1955 Lasker Awards ceremony. (Link family)

11. Warfarin for People

to stay an extra day in New York City after the press luncheon? UW News Service Science Editor James Larsen sent a note to Karl, who replied unenthusiastically. Larsen then wrote back to New York encouraging that Karl be contacted directly. "I am positive he would make an extremely colorful subject for a *Life* article," Larsen wrote. "Just about the most colorful I could think of."

The *Life* article didn't happen. But around the same time, in late September 1955, Karl got a game-changing card from someone with Wisconsin ties working in a military hospital in Colorado.

President Dwight D. Eisenhower, still in his first term, was vacationing in the Denver area and staying at the home of his in-laws. On Sept. 23, Eisenhower played golf at the Cherry Hills Country Club and complained of feeling ill. The next morning, after again complaining of chest pains, an electrocardiogram revealed that the president had suffered a serious heart attack.

Just a few days later, Karl received the card – written from a former Wisconsinite now at the Fitzsimmons Army Hospital in Denver.

"The President is getting one of your drugs and it is not dicumarol," the note read.

Presidential press secretary J. C. Hagerty gave the country a brief update on Eisenhower's condition:

"The heparin which was used initially as the anticoagulant has been replaced by a drug of the dicumarol type. The present prothrombin level has been well maintained."

Karl felt fairly certain Eisenhower was receiving Coumadin. The physician in charge was Fitsimmons cardiologist Colonel Byron Pollock, whose paper titled, "Clinical experience with warfarin (coumadin sodium a new anticoagulant)," had been read at a medical conference in New Jersey and was awaiting publication in the *Journal of American Medicine*.

"I surmised," Karl said later, "that the most important man in the world today was being anti-coagulated via warfarin sodium."

It would, of course, be a tremendous boost of positive publicity if the public learned the President Eisenhower was being treated with warfarin/Coumadin. Yet no official word was given. That led to an anxious letter, written Oct. 6 – two weeks after Eisenhower's heart attack – by Samuel Gordon of Endo Products to Ward Ross, managing director of WARF, with a copy to Karl.

"Dear Ward," Gordon began. "I have been scanning the papers very carefully about the course of our president's illness. We are all terribly disturbed for partisanship does not mix with sickness.

"There are several items which interest us. Colonel Byron E. Pollock, whom I regard as a good friend, is the physician immediately in charge. As you recall, his paper is now awaiting publication by the A.M.A."

Gordon continued: "I would like to believe that all of the talk about coronary thrombosis in the papers will be helpful. You or I might have written either Dr. White's [Paul White, Eisenhower's post-heart attack cardiologist] comments or other items on the condition, which appeared in the papers...

"While I cannot establish it, I have a deep feeling that Colonel Pollock gave Coumadin to the president. It would be heartless if I tried to find out now – if I were so brash as to do it, Colonel Pollock has a right to pin my ears back. But that will come in time.

"Why do I have the feeling that the President was given warfarin?" Gordon concluded. "I spent an afternoon with Colonel Pollock a week before the President's illness. He showed me one case that pretty near paralleled that of the President. Coumadin was given to this patient – it is the only anticoagulant that the Colonel uses at Fitzsimmons. It would have been nice for us if that were mentioned, assuming that my feeling has some base. But we must rest on fact, not on vague hope."

Five weeks later, Gordon wrote another letter to Ross, again copying Karl, on the same topic. Gordon referenced a recent press

11. Warfarin for People

conference by Dr. White where he discussed keeping President Eisenhower on anticoagulants, mentioning both dicumarol and Coumadin.

"This is stronger presumptive evidence than we had before that Coumadin was used," Gordon wrote. "But the mention along with dicumarol does cloud up the picture a bit. Of course, White is talking about coronary thrombosis in general. Dicumarol is at least 13 years old to him – Coumadin is new to him – about 7 weeks at most. It is unlikely that White would say Coumadin if it weren't actually used."

Gordon concluded, "We would like to say the President received Coumadin. All we can say and be bound by the rules of evidence that it is more than probable that the President had Coumadin."

As it turned out, more than a year would pass before the public learned that President Eisenhower had been treated with warfarin/Coumadin.

Fittingly, it was Karl who delivered the news.

In summer 1957, Karl accepted an invitation from his friend and colleague Dr. Irving Wright, in New York City, to attend and speak the following February at the New York Academy of Medicine on the discovery of dicumarol and its sequels.

On Sept. 26, 1957, Wright wrote Karl with some of the details of the February event, which would cover several days and gather many national experts on anticoagulants. Dr. Jay McLean of Johns Hopkins, who discovered the first anti-clotting chemical, heparin, in 1916, would be honored posthumously.

"If you have new findings," Wright wrote Karl, "this will be a fine opportunity to present them for wide coverage."

Karl took full advantage, delivering the Feb. 25 address that has been referenced often in this narrative. He started with the story of farmer Ed Carlson and wove it all the way to a military hospital in Denver in September 1955. Karl mentioned the postcard he'd received about President Eisenhower being treated with one of Karl's drugs "and it's not dicumarol."

Karl said he surmised it was warfarin sodium.

"This surmise proved to be correct," Karl told his New York City audience.

The next day's papers trumpeted the news. "Physicians Laud New Heart Drug," read the headline in the *New York Times*. The article began, "The development of a chemical that is both a powerful rat poison and an anticoagulant was hailed here last night. It has been used by President Eisenhower since shortly after his heart attack in Denver on Sept. 24, 1955."

Newspapers near and far spread the word about Ike and warfarin. Karl's hometown paper, the *Wisconsin State Journal*, had it on page one Feb. 26 with the headline: "Dr. Link's Drug Used on President."

As a footnote to Karl's celebrated lecture, Elizabeth Link, two weeks before Karl spoke in New York, wrote a letter to Dr. Irving Wright, Karl's colleague in working with anticoagulants and the one who invited him to lecture in New York.

"Dear Dr. Wright," Karl's wife wrote. "This is to inform you that Professor Link's manuscript for the 2-25 affair of the New York Heart Association has been posted today.

> *"In the 28 years that I have known Karl, he has heretofore never sent off the manuscript for a lecture before delivering it orally. Indeed he usually drives people mad trying to get him to supply manuscripts. The first time he spoke on dicumarol at the Mayo Clinic in March 1942 they [badgered] him for 6 months trying to get the manuscript. In the meantime he kept on experimenting – and they finally gave up. It was never submitted.*
>
> *So I congratulate you on your success in extracting this one.*
>
> *Cordially yours,*
> *Elizabeth Link"*

On March 3, 1958, Irving Wright wrote Karl a note thanking him for speaking in New York. "It was a very pleasant and stimulating

11. Warfarin for People

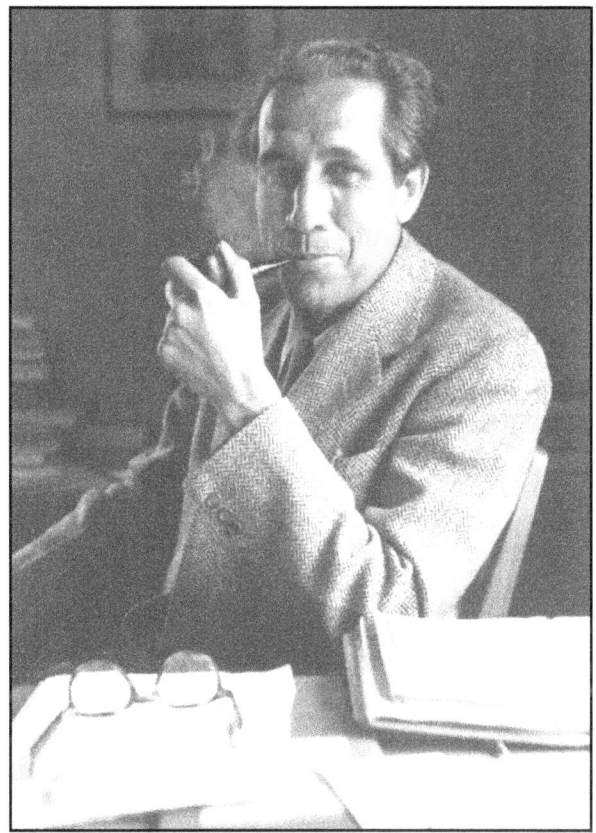

Karl with a pipe and a wry smile. (UW-Madison Archive)

evening and you added immeasurably to this," Wright wrote, encouraging Karl to send a statement with his expenses for the trip.

On May 5, the *State Journal* published a lengthy profile of Karl, a "human interest" piece penned by a friendly reporter, John Newhouse.

Newhouse noted how there were essentially two Karl Paul Links, one known to the world at large, and another known to his fellow Madisonians.

"To the rest of the world," Newhouse wrote, "outside of Madison, he is one of the top scientists of the century – a man who does brilliant work, inspires great work in his research teams and is a leading teacher.

"Here in Madison, however, we're used to seeing him needing a haircut, needing a shoe-shine, driving a beat-up station wagon, and getting into fascinating brawls with eminently respectable persons who have impeccable haircuts and wonderfully well-polished shoes."

Newhouse then catalogued a few of Karl's controversies, including his feud with Steenbock and his off-campus calf scours research. Newhouse mentioned a current effort, in which Karl joined Linus Pauling and others in the United States, Great Britain and the Soviet Union, in "suing their governments to make them stop atomic explosions because of the dangers of fallout."

Newhouse wrote that Karl was "a little concerned that he's mellowing as he grows older." The article closed with Newhouse quoting Karl on "his philosophy":

"Always face life like a pitcher in a ball game, confronting the umpire. All you want is justice, for him to call 'em as you throw 'em. And when you don't get a fair call, treat life the way any good pitcher would treat an umpire. Give it to 'em!"

In September 1958, Karl presided over a celebratory dinner in Chicago for an old friend. Writing about the event later, Karl noted that it started in December of the preceding year, when he shared a train ride with another friend, Sidney Cantor, a carbohydrate chemist who started a chemical consulting company.

The train was late leaving its station. "When the train finally got underway," Karl wrote, "Sid opened a package containing some Herkimer County cheese and kippered herring, whereupon I displayed my briefcase containing several cans of OLD Tankard Ale (Pabst). The conversation ranged far and wide. Finally, a substantial idea appeared to be hatching in Sid's mind."

Cantor said, "You know, the American Chemical Society meets in Chicago the first week in September of 1958 and Carl Miner's 80th birthday is on the 8th of August. Something ought to be done about that. What do you think about having a Carl Miner dinner?"

11. Warfarin for People

Karl didn't hesitate. "You're talking to the self-appointed presider for that occasion."

Miner was a past chairman of the American Chemical Society and sometimes called the "father of furfural chemistry." He founded Miner Laboratories in Chicago in 1906. Later, Miner pulled together a group of grain industry executives and consulting scientists – Karl was one – for a "Starch Round Table" that met to discuss grain-related topics. As journalist Don Behm noted, "Many of Karl's closest friendships were established in the business world as consultant to both government and Midwestern corporations."

The dinner on Sept. 8, 1958, was a great success, as 65 men who had worked with and/or been mentored by Miner came to the Chicago Bar Association on South LaSalle Street to celebrate. Among them was a vice president of Quaker Oats and the research chief at R.J. Reynolds Tobacco.

Karl noted later: "Those who couldn't come, wrote gladly; those who came but were not asked to speak came gladly; and those who spoke, spoke gladly, for they were eager to greet one whose wise and gentle friendship was a special privilege to them all. All knew that Carl Miner had never set out to dominate, but simply be of use."

Miner wrote Karl a note of thanks:

> *"Dear K.P.L.,*
> *"For your unsurpassable operation as chief engineer of the celebration, my heartfelt thanks. Nobody – but nobody – ever had anything more pleasant happen to him. Carl."*

The following month, however, an old adversary reared its head.

Karl, on Oct. 27, 1958, recorded the visit: "The Captain called again last night."

Karl's mention of "The Captain" is a reference to a 17th-century book by John Bunyan, "The Life and Death of Mr. Badman," in which Bunyan notes the fierceness of Karl's foe – tuberculosis – which in Bunyan's time was called consumption.

Bunyan wrote, "The Captain of all these men of death that came against him to take him away, was the consumption, for it was that that brought him down to the grave."

In his biographical memoir of Karl, Don Behm quotes Karl on the disease, in words Behm found written on an inside cover of one of Karl's books: "Like one that on a lonesome road Doth walk in fear and dread And having once turned round, walks on And turns no more his head; Because he knows a frightful fiend, Doth close behind him tread." (Behm doesn't note it, but Karl was quoting Samuel Coleridge's "Rime of the Ancient Mariner.")

Karl's youngest son, five-year-old Paul, also came down with tuberculosis and entered the Morningside Sanitarium in Monona, near Madison. Paul would remain there a year; Karl's bout was less severe and he was released from his stay at Lake View Sanitarium in spring 1959.

On his previous Lake View visit, Karl wrote a sharply critical appraisal of the circumstance at the sanitorium. This time, Behm noted, "his irrepressible gaiety was a most valuable therapy to counter the bedside sadness of many tubercular patients."

Karl did get involved in at least one controversy during his 1958-59 stay at Lake View.

In January 1959, Karl wrote a letter to UW President Conrad Elvehjem asking Elvehjem to oppose plans for a new building in what was called "Bascom Woods," a wooded area between the Carillon Tower and the Elizabeth Waters residence hall. Its eight acres were just about the only remaining forest land on campus, and Karl's impassioned defense of it is indicative of his deep feeling for the natural world.

In his inimitable prose, Karl told Elvehjem, "History will adjudge you as having been either a hero or a bum on this issue."

Unsurprisingly, Karl's letter found its way into the *Wisconsin State Journal.*

While his efforts were not successful – what is now the William H. Sewell Social Sciences Building was built on the site – the opposition of Karl and others, including faculty from the

11. Warfarin for People

Botany Department, led to the establishment of a "Woods Committee" to help preserve campus green space, an effort that eventually morphed into the Lakeshore Nature Preserve Committee that, according to the Social Sciences website, "today oversees policies and long-term stewardship of these precious natural areas."

That same month – January 1959 – when Karl was fighting to preserve the trees on campus, *Circulation*, a journal of the American Heart Association, published his 1958 New York City lecture under the title "The Discovery of Dicumarol and Its Sequels." Also in January Karl was profiled in the American Medical Association's journal *Today's Health* as part of its series "Men Behind the Medical Miracles."

The attention brought Karl correspondence from friends and colleagues around the country.

"The two articles on the adventures of Karl Paul Link are very welcome," wrote future Nobel laureate Stanford Moore from the Rockefeller Institute in New York. "The record presents an impressive challenge for any scholar. The impact that your work has had is so wide that the reader has to stop and ponder for a little while to let the whole significance sink in."

"You have made a contribution to the care of the sick which shall live forever, a privilege which is denied most of us," wrote E.V. Allen from the Mayo Clinic. "Indeed, you have done more than any physician who is alive at the present time in my estimation with the possible exception of those who developed the antibiotics, and you have achieved a secure place in medical history."

E.V. McCollum wrote from Johns Hopkins: "Your investigation of this problem is one of the very finest scientific studies in the history of biochemistry… How can it be that [Henrik] Dam received the Nobel Prize for his investigations of vitamin K, when you have been passed by after contributing new knowledge of about equally great importance in therapy. You should have had the prize. You should have had it a second time for discovering warfarin."

Karl didn't win the Nobel Prize, but in summer 1959, it was announced he'd be receiving the prestigious John Scott Award, which dated to 1816 and was established by a Scottish chemist to honor "ingenuous men who make useful inventions."

The award was presented later that year, at a Dec. 3 dinner at the Simon House, a downtown Madison restaurant. Elizabeth joined Karl at the dinner and what may have been most interesting about it – both Madison daily papers noted it in their headlines about the dinner – was how thankful and gracious Karl was to everyone in attendance, including some university administrators with whom he had sparred in the past.

The *State Journal* headline read: "Link, 'Ex-Bad Boy of Campus,' Takes Award in Mellowed Mood."

"I've been labeled a bad boy of the campus in the past," Karl noted from the podium. "But tonight I'm going to surprise you."

Among those in attendance who Karl thanked were University President Conrad Elvehjem, former president E.B. Fred and WARF, the technology transfer foundation that helped secure patents and was represented by several people at the dinner.

"Let me add," Karl said, "that the success of my work would not have been possible without the help of the foundation."

A few days after the Scott Award dinner, the *Wisconsin State Journal* ran an editorial saluting Karl with a headline that utilized phrasing from the Scott Award: "The 'Useful' Karl Paul Link."

Of the award, the paper noted, "It couldn't have happened to a more deserving person, and Madison should glow with vicarious pride in his accomplishment. Dr. Link has been lucky, hardworking, and shrewd in his accomplishments, furthermore, he is aging well as a Madison character, to boot…"

12. LESS TEACHING AND ANOTHER LASKER

ON FEB. 18, 1960, KARL wrote a letter to the four faculty colleagues who made up the course committee in the UW's Biochemistry Department.

> *"Gentlemen:*
> *Re: Chemistry and Biochemistry 224 (Carbohydrate Chemistry)*
> *"I am herewith suggesting that consideration be given to replacing Link. In keeping with my usual policy I hasten to add that I do not wish to exert any influence on who takes over."*

Karl noted that in 1929 the course was being taught by Professor Richard Fischer, who, on being stricken with arthritis, asked Karl to take his place.

"At that time, I was contributing to carbohydrate literature," Karl wrote. "This is not the situation today. The stream has gone by me. There is perhaps nothing sadder than the artist who attempts to stay on the stage beyond his time."

Karl concluded by saying that after 30 years, he intended to teach the class one more semester, beginning in fall 1960. But within less than six weeks, he had changed his mind.

On April 29, Karl was invited to address 250 UW medical students at the school's annual field day at the Service Memorial Institute's auditorium on Charter Street.

In a career of memorable oratory, this one likely ranks near the top.

Karl began by saying, "This is a day of triumph for me. This is my first public lecture since June 1958," explaining how the return of tuberculosis had slowed him.

"I am by birth a sort of native skeptic," Karl noted, "with a leaning toward the optimistic side."

The next day's *State Journal* reported that Karl's ensuing address was a rousing triumph, with Karl "gesturing, wisecracking, philosophizing [and] heckling the audience."

"After a lengthy salute to the doctors who treated him," the paper noted, "advice on how to ride Europe's Orient Express for second-class fare in a first-class seat, quoting from John Bunyan's 'The Life and Death of Mr. Badman,' Dr. Link assured his chuckling audience, 'Well, the lecture's going to start pretty soon.'"

The balance of his talk retold the dicumarol story, while allowing, "That's common knowledge now. They even know it in Boston."

Karl concluded with some advice for the medical students:

> *"You must ask questions. The right questions come only through sweat and tears. If you have never eaten your scientific bread with tears in your eyes, perhaps pinched by the fear that you are totally wrong, then I grieve for you."*

At the conclusion, the students rose for a standing ovation. But Karl wasn't quite finished. The triumphal march from Verdi's 1871 opera, "Aida," began to play, and the students marched out to it, grinning.

Had Karl been sending a signal? Just three days later, on May 2, 1960, the *Wisconsin State Journal* carried a headline: "Link, Noted UW Scientist, Retires."

He was retiring from teaching, Karl said, not research.

12. Less Teaching and Another Lasker

"I'm too tired," he noted, "and teaching takes too much out of me. I never give the same lecture twice."

The lengthy article summarized Karl's career, hitting highlights like his lab's discoveries of dicumarol and warfarin; noting that he "fought bitterly" with Harry Steenbock and "also did battle with University Pres. Conrad Elvehjem, then dean of the graduate school, over calf-scours research."

It was a typical retirement story for a distinguished member of the community and a proper sendoff – except that Karl wasn't going anywhere, and he wasn't retiring. Not only would his lab work continue, he'd find other areas of interest – conservation was a big one – in which to apply himself.

Meanwhile, there was family news. The previous December, Karl and Elizabeth's oldest son, John Link, got married. The bride was Ruth Bella Lurie, and the couple met while attending undergraduate school at Antioch College in Yellow Springs, Ohio. John later earned a National Sciences Foundation fellowship in theoretical physics at Pasadena's California Institute of Technology – Caltech.

In November 1960, Karl and Elizabeth Link's first grandchild was born to John and Ruth, a daughter named Elisabeth. That welcome news was followed a few months later by a telegram addressed to John Link at his parents' Madison home in the Highlands. Wisconsin's U.S. Sen. William Proxmire was letting John know that his graduate fellowship was being extended to a third year. "Your achievement," Proxmire wrote, "reflects great credit on your community and state as well as your school and is a source of pride to me as your Senator."

In March 1960, Karl lost a valued friend, Bill Olson, who died at 56 in Milwaukee, where he was chairman of the English department at Spencerian College. Olson was a native of Stoughton, just outside Madison, and Karl had met him while both were students at the University of Wisconsin. Olson was studying English and was introduced to Karl in 1927 by William Ellery Leonard, the UW English professor who assisted Karl with the English themes he was struggling with as an undergraduate. It was Olson and his wife or wife-to-be, Rose, who, in 1928, introduced Karl Paul Link and Elizabeth Feldman.

Karl and Madison Rabbi Manfred Swarsensky gave eulogies at Olson's funeral.

Karl's was heartfelt and highly personal, and as is sometimes the case, probably said as much about Karl as it did about Olson.

"Bill and I romanticized many times over those [student] days of the late 1920s," Karl said. "Bill would say, 'Remember that night in June 1928 when we walked out to Picnic Point after that storm in mud up to our shoe tops?' Then he would chuckle. His warm happy chuckle is a thing I have recalled again and again. It was a chuckle of appreciation, understanding and love."

A little later, Karl said, "Bill loved teaching. In his work with young people he tried to find the spark of creativity in each. Many of his students became his loyal friends. Through his influence they became seekers of truth... This love of teaching was part of his love for and faith in men. He retained an optimistic view of man's power to create the Good Life. One quality stands above all others, his warm acceptance and love of his fellow man. He did not judge men. Not even those who had been unjust to him."

A few days later, Rose Olson sent Karl a note.

"Everyone who heard you said that was the best funeral oration they'd ever heard and that the combination of you and Swarsensky was perfect," Rose wrote. "Everyone said they felt healthier and more alive for having been there. That is a rare tribute to both your eloquence and your creativity... It meant more than I can say."

A brief *Capital Times* story on Olson's death and the service gave Karl a chance to show his peevish side – irritation mixed with a bit of humor.

The *Cap Times* article noted that Olson's funeral was officiated by Swarsensky and "Dr. Carl Paul Link of Madison."

12. LESS TEACHING AND ANOTHER LASKER

A day or two later – as related in a note Karl kept among his papers – Karl called the newspaper's editor and publisher, William T. Evjue.

"I told him that I had a complaint to register on his paper, 'The Wright Times.'"

Karl was seemingly poking fun at the reverence afforded Frank Lloyd Wright by both Evjue and his newspaper.

Of his complaint, Karl continued: "To wit: After 32 years of acquaintance with K.P.L. the Wright Times does not know how to spell my name and that I'm not a resident of Madison (town of Middleton, since 1931)."

Karl couldn't get too upset at *The Capital Times* – they provided excellent coverage of Elizabeth Link's extensive, enduring work on behalf of the Women's International League of Peace and Freedom (WILPF), a non-governmental organization

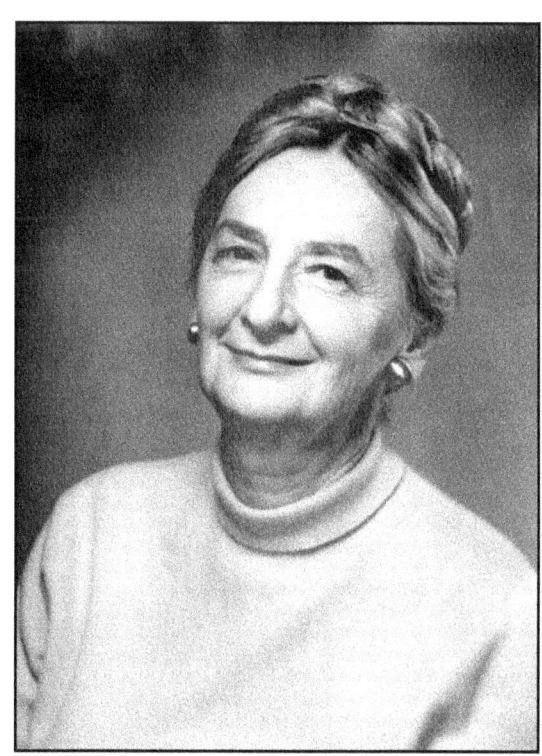

Elizabeth Feldman Link.
(Link family)

that evolved out of the 1919 Second Women's International Congress for Peace and Freedom headed by Jane Addams.

How far back did Elizabeth Link go with the WILPF? Her mother Molly joined the Madison chapter in 1923. In May 1931, newly married to Karl, Elizabeth starred in a UW campus production of a two-actor play called "Mother of Men," described as "a war tragedy" and co-sponsored by the Women's International League.

By 1960, Elizabeth was the Madison chapter president. A year earlier, as chair of the finance committee and co-chair of the legislative committee, Elizabeth spent five days in Washington, D.C. where she visited embassies and lobbied with others in the WILPF to "foment public opinion behind the total cessation of nuclear testing" and the recognition of the legitimacy of communist China.

The year 1960 was the centennial of Jane Addams' birth, and the Madison chapter of the league celebrated with numerous events, many of them held at Elizabeth and Karl's home in the Highlands. In August of that year, Elizabeth and the local chapter helped bring the Rev. Curtis Crawford to Madison, where he spoke on the Capitol Square on the folly of the arms race.

That spring, having retired from teaching – though not research – Karl launched himself at a project that reflected his growing passion for conservation. He decided to develop a better bird food.

Naturally, he invited his reporter friend, John Newhouse, out to the Highlands to discuss it.

"I am a little tired of killing rats," Karl said, and, in a reference to President Eisenhower, added, "and saving politicians' lives. Now I'd like to do something for the feathered denizens of the sky, who give us so much, and ask so little."

The need was there, Karl said. "Cities are getting large. Hedgerows are disappearing, and highways are taking more and more land out of circulation. As a result, it's becoming more and more important to find a low-cost food for birds."

12. Less Teaching and Another Lasker

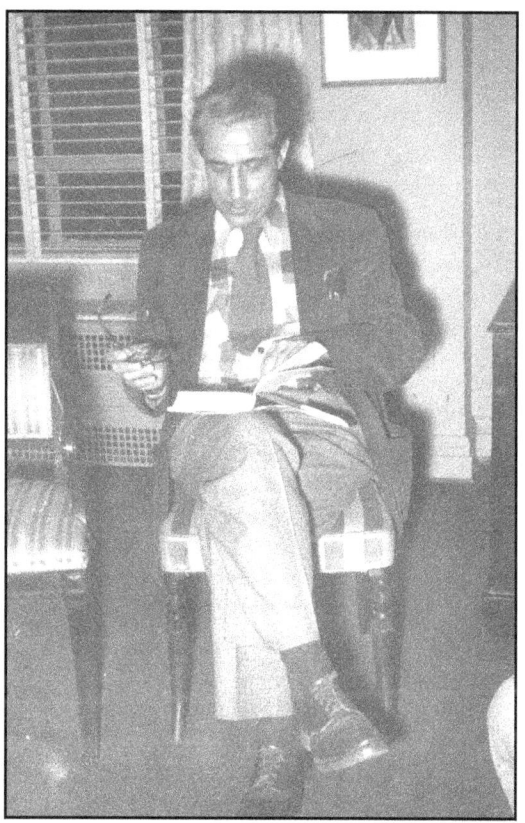

Karl engaged in one of his favorite pastimes. (Link family)

Karl told Newhouse his interest in birds and their feed dated to his childhood in Indiana, when his family was "so poor" that Karl and his brothers were dispatched to the ditches adjacent to the railroad tracks to gather weed seeds for the Link family's canary and warbler.

"They were the healthiest birds in town," Karl said. "There's a lesson to be learned there."

Newhouse noted: "The only problem is that, though he's walked up and down the tracks and talked with all his brothers but the one in Africa and the one in Brazil, he still can't remember one of the weed seeds he collected."

"My job," Karl said, "is to learn what nature has to tell me – not to set up an elaborate theory and then try to muster facts to justify my theory. And where the information nature gives the close observer will lead, no one knows."

Squirrels did not benefit from Karl's engagement with birds, rather they angered him by eating the nutritious bird feed he'd developed.

"I offered them shrimp, and crab, and mushrooms," Karl said of the squirrels. "I tried moose suet, and honey, in and out of the comb. I tried truffles, and coconut, but they were not to be distracted. They preferred my vitalized food to the devitalized concoctions humanity finds so much pleasure in eating."

Karl did find a solution to the squirrel problem: his 1906 single-shot .22 rifle.

A year later, it was not squirrels, but rather the military jets from Truax Field that stirred Karl's ire. He sent a missive to *Capital Times* columnist Herb Jacobs, written, Jacobs noted, "in the best tongue-in-cheek Link style" and addressed to Jacobs in care of "The Wright Times, a newspaper." (Karl knew that not only was *The Capital Times* friendly to Frank Lloyd Wright, the famed architect had designed and built two homes for Herb Jacobs, a personal friend.)

"What's the law on how low these playboys can fly over the city of Madison?" Karl asked. "And at what hours of the day they can play over Madison's skies?

"As you know, the Highlands is mostly in the city of Madison. The Link bird haven is still in the town of Middleton, but it's nearly surrounded by the city.

"These jet-playboys scare my birds away!"

Jacobs dutifully contacted a UW professor of wildlife, who would not have endeared himself to Karl with this quote: "The whole history of aviation is that birds become accustomed to tremendous noises."

Eugene Roark, who edited a Wisconsin bird magazine called *The Passenger Pigeon*, took Karl's bird work more seriously. Roark wrote a piece for the winter 1961-62 issue of *Wisconsin Tales and Trails* magazine titled, "Medicine for Man, Poison for

12. Less Teaching and Another Lasker

Pests, and a Better Bird Seed" that highlighted Karl's recent bird adventures. It makes the point that Karl was ahead of his time in being leery of the wholesale use of chemical agents in nature.

"Dr. Link is concerned about the future of birds," Roark wrote, "in a country which seems to be cleaning up its backyards, farm hedgerows and parks, removing the brush and weeds where birds find both food and nesting places. He's alarmed by the amount of weed killers and insect sprays, and the damage they may do to plants and insects upon which birds depend – and to birds themselves."

In December 1962, the Link family home in La Porte, Indiana was the subject of a two-page color spread in *House and Garden* magazine. Karl's brother Alfred continued to live in the home and decorated the Christmas tree each year in such a glorious fashion that *House and Garden* used it to inaugurate a "Most Splendid Christmas Tree Competition."

Karl would recall that some of the ornaments on the tree were already 40 years old when he was a boy. *House and Garden* wrote: "The most wonderful, truly for Christmas tree H and G has ever seen is this one, a family affair that comes to life each year under the La Porte, Ind. roof of Judge Alfred J. Link, an insatiable collector of Christmas tree memorabilia. One of his earliest acquisitions, a cocky glass bird, still spends the month required to trim the tree as a watchman wired to the living room chandelier. For almost fifty years, this glassy old fellow has been the Christmas bird."

As noted, though Karl retired from teaching in 1960, he didn't leave his lab. Proof of his ongoing importance in the scientific community came in summer 1960 with a letter informing Karl he'd won a second Lasker Award from the American Heart Association (his first was in 1955). This time, he shared the honor – often referred to as the "American Nobel Prize" – with two distinguished friends and colleagues, Dr. Irving Wright of Cornell University and Dr. Edgar V. Allen of the Mayo Clinic. They were cited for their work with anticoagulants, and each

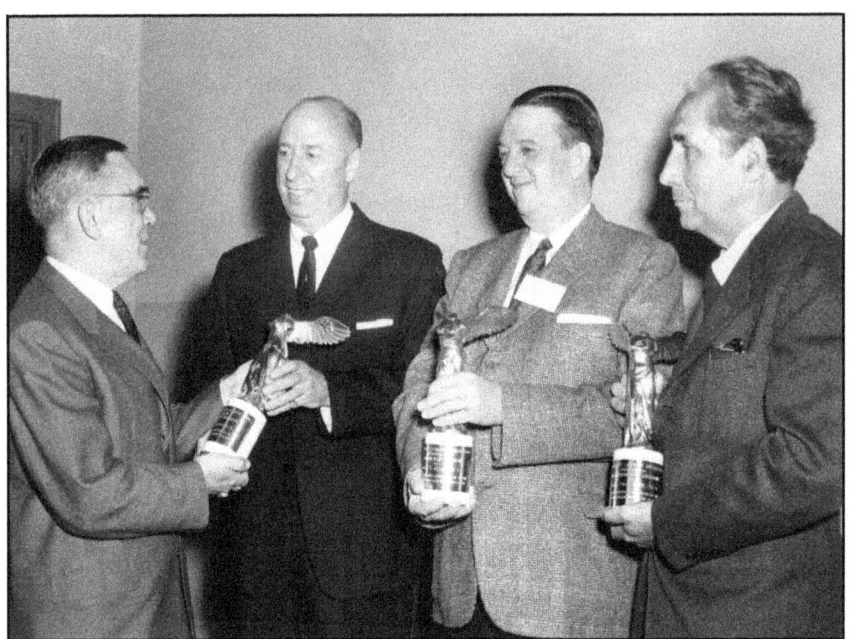

Karl, far right, shown receiving the prestigious Lasker Award for his scientific achievements. He was one of a handful of two-time recipients. (Link family)

received $2,500, an illuminated scroll and a gold statuette of the Winged Victory of Samothrace, symbolizing victory over death and disease.

Karl was the second individual to receive two Lasker Awards (as of summer 2020, there were six). First – having received the award in 1954 and 1959 – was Robert Gross, a pioneering cardiac surgeon.

In July 1960, Karl received a note from Mary Lasker, widow of Albert Lasker, whose fortune allowed the couple to endow the awards. They'd married in 1940, by which time Albert was recognized as an advertising genius, the country's first. He expanded outside the advertising business with endeavors that included an early ownership of the Chicago Cubs. According to the 2010 biography, "The Man Who Sold America," Lasker also suffered from a form of what is now known as bipolar disorder, which may have given him something else in common with Karl

12. Less Teaching and Another Lasker

Paul Link. (In his later years, those close to Karl noted more frequent manic-depressive tendencies.) Lasker's biographer wrote, "He was frequently expansive, irritable, highly verbal, intensely creative and insomniac."

When Lasker died in 1952, Mary Lasker was determined to keep the awards, founded in 1945, going. Indeed, many feel they were her idea, stemming from her experiences at the University of Wisconsin – she grew up in Watertown – during the 1918 flu epidemic. She came to believe fervently in medical research and helped convince the federal government to get involved. Dr. Jonas Salk called her "a matchmaker between science and society."

Mary Lasker's July 5, 1960 note to Karl read: "I am delighted that the Heart Association wishes to give you another Lasker Award. I am not sure whether or not they were aware of the fact that you had already received one Award, but the work is so important that I think it is a good idea for you to be honored again with Irving Wright and E.V. Allen."

Karl wrote a gracious reply to Mary Lasker, in which he humorously suggested "my third award" should go to Dr. Ovid Meyer of the University of Wisconsin Medical School.

Karl felt strongly that Meyer's clinical contribution to the successful development of anticoagulants should be recognized. Karl made the point in his response to a Nov. 2, 1960, letter from Dean William S. Middleton, chief medical director of the Veterans Administration in Washington. Middleton had sent Karl a question about whether rats might be gaining resistance to warfarin, at the same time congratulating Karl on the Lasker honor.

"Apropos the Lasker Award," Karl wrote Middleton, "I wish to indicate that the American Medical Association has given me all the recognition that I deserve. The best recognition after all is the use to which the profession has put our work – and this while I am alive.

"This Lasker Award would have pleased me much more," Karl continued, "had Ovid Meyer been recognized for his basic work with dicumarol, etc. From my point of view, omitting Ovid is not a fair deal within the medical circle. We must concede that 'promoters' are entitled to their dues. But not, as I see it, until the basic clinician is recognized.

"I indicated this point of view to various doctors at St. Louis [the awards were presented Oct. 22 at an American Heart Association function in Missouri] though one is not supposed to look at the teeth of a gift horse."

As for warfarin resistance, Karl noted, "To date we have no evidence that rats are acquiring resistance to warfarinized baits when the warfarin is at the recommended... level. The limiting factor is not the warfarin, but the palatability of the food used as its carrier, how much warfarinized food is available, and where it is placed... By keeping at the job I have never had a failure."

Among those sending congratulatory notes to Karl on the Lasker honor was Donald Slichter, president of the Northwestern Mutual Life Insurance Company and son of the late Charles Slichter, once dean of the UW Graduate School and an early booster of Karl's.

"I well recall the enthusiastic predictions that Father made years and years ago about the contributions that a young graduate student by the name of Link would make to science,' Donald Slichter wrote. "How right he was! We alumni of the University have great cause to be proud of your outstanding achievements in Biochemistry and the great assistance that you have been to mankind."

Karl also received friendly Lasker congratulations from Carl Steiger, a member of the UW Board of Regents, a group with which Karl did not always enjoy amiable relations. Earlier that year, Steiger sent Karl a note on his winning the Scott Award, and Karl sent an unusually personal response, handwritten, in which he noted that he was not retiring, only stepping aside from lecturing, which Karl called "preaching."

"I ended up with what MDs call 'preacher's throat after the April 29 sermon,'" Karl wrote Steiger. "I had been holding

12. Less Teaching and Another Lasker

communion on it for about two months as is revealed in letters to those concerned... I felt lower than the underside of a turtle stuck in the mud the day after I indicated that I had to quit 'preaching.' But I'm getting over that grief. Believe me if you knew how I love to hear myself talk you would understand why I felt so low."

Still, Karl told Steiger, "I am feeling right well these days, and enjoying life." He then quoted Oliver Wendall Holmes: "Life is a great experiment."

In 1961, Karl brought a graduate student named Walt Barker into his lab, and Barker, along with several of Karl's late-career students, would work to solve the remaining mysteries of warfarin, including how it metabolized in a rat. Clearly, it caused the rat to bleed internally, but how and why?

Barker was a chemistry graduate from Purdue University and first came to Madison in 1959 to further his study in that field.

"It just wasn't going well," Barker said, recalling his first two years at UW. "It didn't feel right."

Barker began asking others on campus about possible alternative fields of study. "Someone suggested I go talk to Dr. Link," Barker said.

Barker made an appointment to meet Karl in his corner office on the second floor of the Biochemistry building.

"I walked in and he asked if I knew anything about him," Barker recalled. "I was embarrassed but I had to say I really didn't."

Karl was unfazed.

"We got to talking," Barker said. "He asked me if I had any hobbies and somehow or other I mentioned that sometimes I liked to repair clocks that weren't working."

Karl, Barker said, jumped at that.

"How do you repair them?" Karl asked. "How do you clean them? Do you just swish them around some, or what?"

"Oh, no," Barker replied. "I take them apart and clean the bearings and put them back together. Sometimes it works."

Karl stepped over to a bookcase on which sat a clock that had stopping running.

"Why don't you take this home and if you get a chance work on it and drop it back off," Karl said.

They then got down to business, and Karl agreed to take Barker on as one of his students.

"I worked that summer at the Enzyme Institute," Barker said, "then moved to Biochemistry in fall 1961."

Barker did fix Karl's clock. "As a matter of fact, I still have it," he said, six decades later. "He gave it to me. It stopped working a long time ago."

Barker recalled that Karl didn't come to the lab every day but was usually seen at least a few times a week. He mentioned Karl's mood swings, more pronounced by the early 1960s, and said the days when Karl didn't come in, he may have been battling depression.

"Other times," Barker said, "when he came in, holy cow, he was like a ball of fire."

Barker loved Karl's lab. "As a matter of fact," he said, "I didn't want to leave. After I got my Ph.D., he hired me for a short time as a post-doc, I think mostly out of generosity. Finally, he told me, 'Walt, you've got to get a job.' I grudgingly said, 'OK. I'll try to find one.'"

Of the science, Barker recalled, "My project was the metabolism of warfarin in a rat. No one knew what happened except for the bleeding. They didn't understand what happened to the molecule in the rat."

A February 1962 story in *The Capital Times* offered this description:

"It is known that Warfarin goes to the liver and interferes with the process of manufacturing prothrombin, but the exact mechanism is unknown. Prothrombin is a protein necessary for blood clotting.

"The Wisconsin scientists are now studying the intermediary metabolism of ingested Warfarin, that is, what chemicals the body

12. Less Teaching and Another Lasker

makes out of it, where they go, and how long they last. This is being done by using a Geiger counter to trace the path of radioactive Warfarin through the bodies of rats."

Barker recalled that Karl enjoyed his reputation as a "character" on the Madison campus. "He reveled in it," Barker said. "He and [department secretary] Ann Terrio would get into arguments. One day, Link brought in a big bag of rhubarb from his garden, dropped it on her desk, and said, 'Here, Ann. Eat this. It's good for your bowels.'"

Barker heard stories during his time in Madison that spoke to Karl's progressive, anti-authoritarian bent. "He was a very liberal person," Barker said. "I heard from numerous sources that during the McCarthy era, he had a couple of FBI agents in his class. He introduced them to the students one morning. I bet they cringed. Before he started the lecture, he said, 'I'd like to introduce you to the two FBI agents up there in the corner.'"

Barker continued: "One of his things with me was he would come into the lab and say, 'Walt, a chemist should be able to do anything.' And I knew I was going to get an outside job. He'd bring in something he wanted repaired or want me to come out to the house and do something for him. But I really kind of liked that. I was out there frequently. I actually took care of the house when he and Elizabeth were away. I took care of his dogs during that time, too."

Like numerous of Karl's students, Barker grew close to him. "I felt like I was a member of his family," Barker said. He recalled later taking his wife and kids to visit at the Highlands home. It was at a time when Karl was not supposed to be eating salt and at one point they walked in on Karl and Walt's daughter eating olives out of a jar in the kitchen. "Our daughter loves olives," Barker said. "Elizabeth wasn't happy."

Barker concluded: "I really liked that man. I thought the world of him. I've often told people there were three men who made a real difference in my life, and he was one of them."

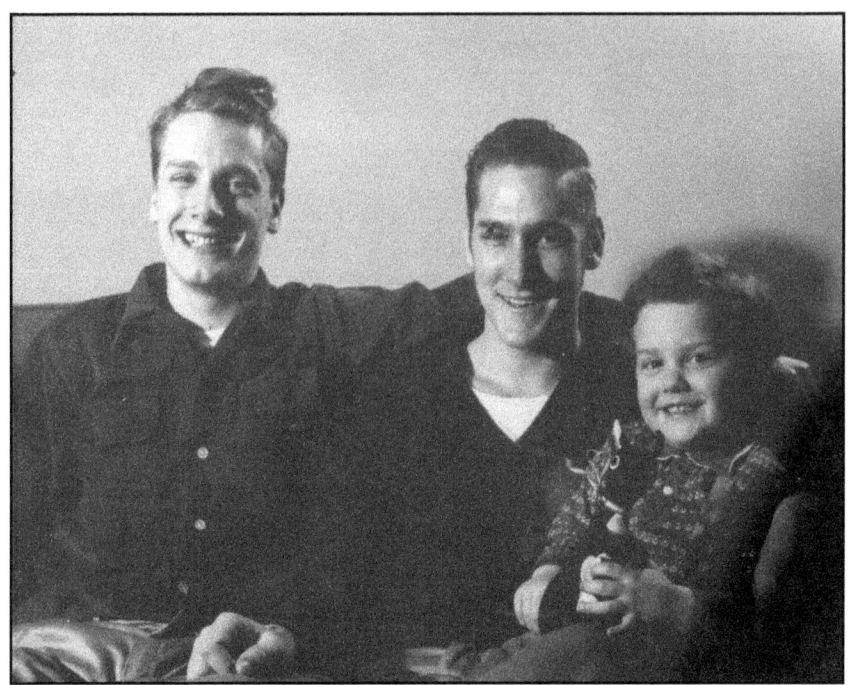

Tom, John, and Paul Link, circa 1957. (Link family)

Campus administrators continued to have their ups and downs with Karl into the 1960s. On May 7, 1962, Karl got a parking ticket he felt he did not deserve, and immediately sent a letter to A. W. Peterson, vice president of business and finance at UW-Madison, expressing his displeasure.

"Dear Al," Karl began. "Were it not for the fact that Connie [Conrad Elvehjem] is already over-burdened with problems that he did not create, can't solve, etc., I would direct this matter to him. Though it is still too hot and humid for May in the state whose motto is FORWARD, I can still show mercy for the distressed and harassed."

Then Karl got to the point.

"When a guy pays 36 bucks a year to park in a lot that is over-assigned, and badly designed, also poorly supervised from the standpoint of the way the cars are parked, usually full of snow in the winter, dirty, dusty, wind-swept, also treeless – (a little shade would help these days), he is forced to push his pencil in

12. LESS TEACHING AND ANOTHER LASKER

protest... Officer No. 8 must have been loitering in lot 30 with a stopwatch in hand between 9 and 11 a.m. I regard this citation as actionable."

Karl signed the letter as follows: "Karl Paul Link, a professor with some mileage behind him – not paid for by the taxpayers of this notorious state – nor charged to WARF. KPL has lost the mellowness reported in the local papers in December 1959 [when he received the Scott Award]. It has been washed out of his body – soul – and spirits by the recent goings-on extant on campus."

Peterson, perhaps deciding discretion in this instance was indeed the better part of valor, sent a note, copying Karl, to UW Protection and Security.

"Gentlemen," Peterson began. "I enclose one dollar in currency in payment of Citation No. 137136 – Professor Karl Paul Link – dated May 7, 1962."

A year later, spring 1963, Karl and Elizabeth and their youngest son, Paul, flew to the Pacific Northwest for second son Tom Link's graduation from Reed College in Portland. The third and oldest brother, John Link, joined them with his wife Ruth and their daughter, Lisa, age 2. Both Tom and John were continuing their educations: Tom had received a fellowship in the Biochemistry Department at Stanford and earned a Ph.D; while John, having received a Ph.D. from Caltech, received a post-doctoral fellowship at the University of California-Berkeley.

In Portland, Karl and Elizabeth spent time with old Madison friends Dr. J. Alfred Hall and his wife, Hall having been director of the Forest Products Lab in Madison. Before they returned to Madison, Tom drove Karl, Elizabeth, and Paul across the border to Victoria, British Columbia to visit Karl's geologist brother, Ted, and his wife Viola.

It's worth noting that Ted Link was regarded as a celebrity in Victoria, where he settled in retirement. In 1964, a year after Karl's family visited, the Victoria newspaper *The Daily Colonialist* published a sprawling profile of Ted titled, "The Man Who Discovered Leduc," a reference to Ted's leading an expedition that found oil riches underground in Alberta.

In mid-January 1964, Karl traveled to Rochester, Minn. for the 12th annual Symposium on Blood Coagulation. Ken McCracken, a staff writer for the *Rochester Post-Bulletin*, reached out and Karl agreed to meet him for an interview at a Rochester hotel coffee shop – at 7 a.m.

"I often get up at 4 a.m. to do my work and go for a walk," Karl told the reporter, adding that he'd taken a pre-dawn stroll around Rochester. "I often take a nap in the afternoon or go to bed right after supper. But then I'm up in the early hours of the morning working on projects."

Many noted that Karl could charm the birds from the trees when he cared to, and McCracken got the full treatment. "A warm, friendly person who lists many unique distinctions," McCracken wrote.

Karl doffed the Tam o' Shanter cap he'd acquired 40 years earlier in Scotland, ordered "two four-minute eggs" and "ran strong fingers through his thick, wavy, almost totally gray hair and reminisced... his brown eyes twinkling behind horn-rimmed glasses."

Of the Link family, Karl told McCracken, "We all are a bunch of individualists and very outspoken."

Of his research, Karl said, "We are just at the frontier of our work," adding that for every success, "there have been 99 failures." Karl said he'd like to help find drugs to combat rheumatoid arthritis and hypertension.

"The entire field is exciting," Karl said. "No one knows what the future holds or what doors will be opened. But the challenge is great, stimulating and the rewards worthwhile and satisfying to the intellect."

Karl was feeling less generous later that month when, in a Jan. 25 letter to Robert Burris, chairman of the UW Biochemistry Department, he pointed out his annual salary and compared it to the $27,500 being awarded to the new Elvehjem professorship in the department. Karl's annual salary increased from $10,200 in 1950 to $17,310 in 1963.

12. Less Teaching and Another Lasker

"I have been hard at it during this period," Karl wrote Burris, "including the six months at Lake View, Oct.-May '58-59. The patent record at WARF will attest to that. How do you suppose I feel when I heard 27-28 grand for the Elvehjem professorship...?

"I have been here since 1927.

"The emphasis has been on quality, in both research and teaching.

"Look at the record.

"Take a look at what you can see on page 744 of the Mayo book on Peripheral Vascular Diseases.

"Look at page 1 of the recent International Anticoagulant Symposium held in Miami Beach, Florida.

"See what kind of impression I made at Rochester, Minn., Jan. 17-18, '64.

"This past summer when the papers carried the large increases many commented, 'I didn't see the name of KPL.' My reply was, 'I'm just a work-horse professor, and apparently I'm not highly regarded by the party.'"

"But ------------- ??!!"

"I'll see you later on this.

"Cordially,

"Karl Paul Link."

Karl could still be feisty, as his colleagues at WARF were soon to be reminded.

13. DOING GOOD FOR MANKIND

A FRONT-PAGE, ABOVE-THE-FOLD headline in the Sunday, Sept. 13, 1964, *Wisconsin State Journal* read:

"10-Year Secret Told: Prof. Link Has New Invention; Way to Bring Rats Home for Kill."

Given its prominent placement in the Sunday (the week's biggest) newspaper, this story – about Karl's discovery of an attractant that would make rats even more susceptible to warfarin – would seem to signal significant scientific news.

Yet the tone of the article, written by Karl's friend and favorite reporter John Newhouse, was almost jocular.

It began: "Thanks to a publisher's garbage can, Prof. Karl Paul Link is coming up with a new invention… The Pied Piper of Hamelin, says Dr. Link, was a good man in his time. But he had to wander about to make the rats follow him. Dr. Link will summon the rats to his poison. Standing still."

Newhouse quoted Karl: "My notes on the rat attractant are labeled 'The Garbage Can Case.' The idea came to me when I was inspecting the garbage can of Don Anderson, publisher of the *Wisconsin State Journal*, on Nov. 24, 1949. Mr. Anderson was suffering from rats. I cannot reveal what I found in the garbage can of Mr. Anderson.…

"I've been working 10 years for this day. I've been keeping secret the work that I've been doing. Now it is beginning to come to light."

Karl's love-hate relationship with WARF also factored in the Newhouse story. Karl noted that the "basic patents" on warfarin were set to expire within days, with negative financial

13. Doing Good for Mankind

implications for WARF. The expiration day the following week, Karl said, was known to WARF managing director Ward Ross as "Black Wednesday."

Karl said he would come to the rescue. "On Thursday," he said, "which shall be known as 'Sunny Thursday' in WARF circles, I shall march into Ross' office and lay on his desk the results of 10 years of work in perfecting the material which will bring rats… to the poison. The smiles will return to his face."

On Sept. 16, three days after the article's publication, Ross sent a letter to all the trustees on the WARF board. His facial expression on composing it may not have been a broad smile.

"Enclosed is a Xerox copy of an article dealing with Dr. Link and WARF which appeared in the *Wisconsin State Journal* Sunday, Sept. 13," Ross wrote.

"This is a typical 'Link type' article and in fact was based on one of Dr. Link's 'press conferences' with John Newhouse of the *State Journal*. While there is considerable humor in the article, at the same time it contains quite a bit of meat.

"The reaction to this article varied greatly. Most employees of the Foundation were quite irritated. Others took the article in good stride and not too seriously.

"It will be of great interest to hear the reactions of the Trustees to this controversial article when we can discuss the matter at the Sept. 26 meeting of the Trustees in Milwaukee."

Karl received a copy of the Ross letter, and on Sept. 18, wrote a succinct appraisal on it in pencil: "This letter stinks."

A week later, Karl spoke with Ross, a meeting the WARF managing director detailed in a Sept. 25 memorandum he titled "Link (Secret) Rodenticide Invention."

Ross wrote: "On Sept. 24, 1964, I proposed to Professor Link that a testing program be initiated for Link's new…rat baits. He flatly refused to have these baits tested by the WARF laboratory under any conditions, and also refused to submit these baits for field trials by WARF personnel. He likewise refused to disclose to me any test data on these baits, Link taking the position that WARF, in regard to the matter of efficacy, 'must take his word for it.'"

Ross concluded, "Link stated that he did not believe his invention should be the subject of a patent, but rather that it be maintained as a trade secret. I advised him that there would be difficulty in having claims proved by Federal regulatory agencies without appropriate test data, but he said that the only claim that need be made is 'a stable and attractive bait.'

"In view of the lack of a complete disclosure and particularly Link's unwillingness to submit his baits to any test program by government, by WARF, or by others, it is obvious there is nothing further WARF can or should do at this time with respect to this development."

It was an odd episode that seems to have gone no further: At least there was no further mention of the "Garbage Can Case" in the press. That it was not completely frivolous on Karl's part can be seen in a 1961 letter, included with his papers, from Karl to a Washington, D.C. patent lawyer named L. D. Dibble.

"I can get an affidavit," Karl wrote, "on the original use under a garbage can from Don Anderson, the [*State Journal*] publisher, to cover the 1949-50 trials on his premises."

Nor should anyone be surprised to learn that after the 1964 Newhouse story in the *State Journal*, Karl began referring to himself as a "master baiter."

He was, in any case, still doing science. In 1964, Karl took on a new graduate student, Mark Hermodson.

"Link was an impressive guy when you met him," Hermodson recalled, in an interview more than half a century later. "He was 63, and a very dynamic guy, full of good humor, very engaging, flamboyant, with a big loud voice."

Hermodson grew up on a Minnesota farm and attended St. Olaf College in that state. He studied chemistry. Upon graduating, Hermodson applied to California-Berkeley and UW-Madison for graduate school. He was accepted by both but was more impressed by the responsiveness of Wisconsin; he enrolled there and passed a qualifying exam that allowed him to move directly into the doctorate program.

Hermodson enjoyed the Link lab. "What I did when I started in the lab was pick up the end of a project Walt Barker had about two-thirds finished," Hermodson said. "It was determining how warfarin is handled in the body of a rat, how it gets metabolized."

Hermodson recalled that after he had been in the lab for a time, Karl obtained "a half dozen warfarin resistant" rats from the United Kingdom, and Hermodson began working on what caused this resistance.

Like other students, especially in later years, Hermodson experienced Karl's bipolar tendencies.

"It appeared almost seasonal," Hermodson recalled. "When I was there, when the weather started to warm up in the spring, he would be in one of his manic moods. There would be notes on the blackboard in the lab: 'Link here. 2 a.m. Where is everybody?'

"During those periods he was just crazy," Hermodson continued. "He would say crazy things. He was minimally cautious about what he said at any time, but during the manic time…"

Once the heat of mid-summer descended, "you wouldn't see him for several weeks and he was really down in the dumps."

Recalling Karl in the lab, Hermodson said, "He wanted to know what you were doing, and as long as he thought you were headed down the right path, it was up to you. He gave an enormous amount of freedom. As a Ph.D. student you have to make that transition from being a recipient of teaching to actually directing your own science."

Though Karl was ostensibly retired from teaching, Hermodson remembered him teaching one class, and teaching it well.

"It was on how to give a decent scientific seminar," Hermodson said. "He was really good at that. He really wanted students to learn how to be engaging. They didn't have to be as flamboyant as he was. But he was good at making sure students could get up and talk in a coherent way and give a decent scientific seminar."

Hermodson said, "I never had anything but good things to say about him."

Hermodson had one more lasting memory, from summer 1965: "I distinctly remember a day when he came in looking downcast in the morning, with the morning newspaper in his hand. It had the news that Adlai Stevenson had dropped dead on the streets of London. Link just shook his head and said, 'The good guys die young. The bastards live forever.'"

In 1964, the year before Stevenson's death, Karl took an active role in the effort to keep Republican Sen. Barry Goldwater from winning the presidency. Karl cochaired – with Marshfield physician Ben Lawton and UW Graduate School Associate Dean Gerard Rohlich – the Wisconsin chapter of the group Scientists, Engineers and Physicians for [Lyndon] Johnson-[Hubert] Humphrey, the Democratic ticket.

A few days before the November 1964 election, Karl, upset with the number of pro-Goldwater letters printed in the *Wisconsin State Journal*, wrote a letter of his own to Madison's morning paper:

"I congratulate the Wisconsin State Journal for its good sense in not supporting Sen. Barry Goldwater, but you'd never know it from your Morning Mail.

"As you know, this is the first time in my life I have joined any kind of political movement, and I am not alone. This campaign has brought a remarkable innovation in American politics – the active participation of many of America's most distinguished scientists, who along with me, are expressing themselves for the first time. And it isn't an accident."

Karl quoted Dr. George Kistiakowsky, science advisor to former President Eisenhower, and "a Republican by the way":

"We believe that Sen. Goldwater is outside the mainstream of responsible American thinking and is clearly unqualified to be trusted with the great powers of the American presidency."

Karl concluded: "Scientists, Engineers, and Physicians for Johnson-Humphrey – bipartisan – have groups in all 50 states and membership of more than 100,000."

13. Doing Good for Mankind

Karl's letter was printed the day before Johnson swamped Goldwater, winning election by roughly 61-39 percent of the popular vote.

If his 1964 support of Johnson – or more accurately, his disdain for Goldwater – marked Karl's entrance into electoral politics, it was not, by any means, his first public engagement with the issues of the day. Karl's willingness to take a stand on such matters defined him as much as anything other than his science.

Examples abound. His work with the Labor Youth League on the UW-Madison campus was covered at length earlier in this narrative. Halting atomic and nuclear proliferation was another passion.

In April 1958, Karl traveled to Washington, D.C. as part of a group – led by his friend Linus Pauling – that filed a lawsuit seeking to block American atomic bomb tests. Similar suits were eventually filed in Great Britain and the Soviet Union.

By then, Karl's activism with Pauling, recipient of the 1954 Nobel Prize in Chemistry (and, later, the Nobel Peace Prize), dated back at least a decade. In 1949, Pauling, then on the faculty at the California Institute of Technology and president of the American Chemical Society, asked Karl to sign onto a letter from the Committee for Peaceful Alternatives to the Atlantic Pact that was delivered to President Harry Truman. The letter asked that steps be taken to outlaw further use of the atomic bomb. Karl agreed to sign.

After filing the lawsuit in Washington in April 1958, the group held a well-attended press conference. Pauling spoke, as did a Connecticut housewife named Stephanie May, who had her two-year-old son with her.

"There is Strontium-90 [radioactive fallout] in the bones of my baby," May said. "It's illegal for someone to put it there when I don't want it there."

Pauling had noted that Strontium-90 was nonexistent prior to the explosion of the first atomic bomb in 1945.

A report on the press conference in the *Baltimore Sun* claimed the "most passionate of the complainants is Karl Paul Link, professor of biochemistry at the University of Wisconsin, introduced by Pauling as discoverer of an anticoagulant used on President Eisenhower after his heart attack."

The *Sun* story then noted: "Link explained that he was an 'agriculturist' who extracted the medication from 'spoiled sweet clover hay,' but his appearance was that of a poet, with a heavy shock of iron-gray hair bulging out like a lion's mane."

The *Sun* reporter then quoted Karl: "I am naïve enough to say before hard-boiled reporters that one reason for my good success was that I tried to do mankind good rather than destroy it. I regard fallout as evil and in the long fight against evil good will win."

His activism continued apace into the next decade: Less than a week after Lyndon Johnson's victory in the November 1964 presidential election, Karl was one of 84 members of the UW-Madison faculty to sign a petition sent to Johnson and the U.S. Department of Justice asking for federal protection for civil rights workers in Mississippi.

In May 1965, Karl was one of five UW scientists honored at a Wisconsin Idea Theater conference in Madison. By then, of course, Karl was not a stranger to awards and accolades, but given his respect for the arts – good writing in particular – the theater's honor must have resonated with him.

Idea Theater head Robert E. Gard noted: "For the first time in the history of the American theater, a statewide theater organization is making an effort to bring science and art closer together. Science is having the greatest boom in history and the living theater is at its highest peak. Since both theater and science are important to the human race, perhaps each can better understand and enjoy the other." The dinner was May 13 at the Park Motor Inn on Madison's Capitol Square.

Ten days after the dinner, the House Committee on Un-American Activities (HUAC) began a series of hearings in

13. Doing Good for Mankind

Chicago on alleged Communist activities in the area. The controversial committee drew protests, including a group of students from the University of Wisconsin – enough protesters that 200 Chicago police officers were assigned to guard the building where the hearings were held.

In Madison, Karl opened an anti-HUAC meeting the evening of May 24 which drew dozens of people to the University YMCA.

The *Capital Times* reported that Karl "demanded that Red-hunters take their allegations into the courts and not make them in the newspapers or on the radio."

On June 9, 1965, Karl wrote a letter of condolence to Dr. Joseph Gale, whose wife of 36 years, Marion, had died unexpectedly while vacationing with her husband in Hawaii. Gale was a University of Wisconsin Hospital surgeon who pioneered the use of resection surgery to help tuberculosis patients, something Karl would have been likely to appreciate.

Karl wrote Gale that he had gone to Rennebohm's Drug Store for a sympathy card. Not finding one to his liking, he sent a letter, which, Karl being Karl, included kind words about the late Mrs. Gale while offering some insight into the man who sent it.

"My pen does not move readily," Karl wrote Gale, at 4:15 a.m. on June 9, 1965. "I hate death." (Karl underlined those three words.) "I find it difficult to attend funerals or visit hospitalized friends.

"What a jolt It must have been to lose Mrs. Gale so suddenly while in that Garden of the Pacific Ocean. But I hasten to add… we should be thankful that when the final call came, she did not have to suffer much. Under such circumstances the final crossing is harder on the survivors than the voyager.

"Mrs. Gale is in my memory since the fall of 1933," Karl wrote. "I met her through our neighbor who brought her to our house while the interior was just a shell. It was a warm beautiful day in early November. I showed her through. She climbed a ladder to the second floor and with my field glasses [appreciated] the beauty of our view. I said to myself, 'You too are beautiful.'

"She was always sweet to me," Karl concluded, and mentioned having last seen her in late August 1964, when she smiled and remarked on his hat.

"It was an old Stetson straw, bought in 1932. I felt happier than usual after the exchange and that last call. With best wishes, in which Mrs. Link joins me."

Elizabeth Link was traveling that summer, helping advance peace-related causes.

In July 1965, Elizabeth flew to the Hague in the Netherlands to attend the Jubilee Congress of the Women's International League for Peace and Freedom. The Congress celebrated the 50th anniversary of the organization's founding (at the Hague) in 1915. Elizabeth, of course, was a past president of the Madison chapter, as was her traveling companion, Mrs. Chester Graham, who was also one of ten United States delegates to the conference, which had delegates from 20 countries.

After the conference, Elizabeth stopped in England, where one of her cousins, Baset Gillinson, an architect, was building a shopping center inspired by those beginning to appear in the United States.

In early 1966, Elizabeth flew to California, for a visit with son Tom, studying for a doctorate in biochemistry at Stanford, and to welcome a new grandchild, named Andrea, born to son John and his wife Ruth. Elizabeth got back to Madison in time for Karl's birthday on Jan. 31 – his 65th – which they celebrated with a dinner at Elizabeth's mother's home on Midvale Boulevard.

Elizabeth's activism included writing a March 1966 letter to *The Capital Times* complimenting the U.S. Senate Foreign Relations Committee for holding hearings on the war in Vietnam. Elizabeth decried the lack of information provided the general American public about the war, noting: "No one who watched… could escape the tremendous sense of urgency that pervaded the whole session… the great historic importance of the hearings, as perhaps the last chance of reaching the American people – over the head of the President – in order to inform them that if our

13. Doing Good for Mankind

present policy continues it will lead the U.S. and the whole world to nuclear war." History tells us that if it didn't do that precisely, the war's escalation in the coming years would prove devastating to the Vietnamese and the tens of thousands of young Americans who lost their lives.

In the late 1960s and early '70s, Elizabeth would attend antiwar protests at the Capitol in Madison, bringing along with her grandchildren and waving origami peace cranes. (She would also march against the proliferation of nuclear weapons and in solumn commemoration of the bombs dropped on Hiroshima and Nagasaki.)

That February, Karl sent a check for $1,000 to an old friend and associate: Eugen Schoeffel, who as a graduate student was present in Karl's laboratory on the fateful day in 1933 when a northern Wisconsin farmer showed up with a bucket of cow's blood. The visit launched Karl's work with anticoagulants. It could hardly have been more consequential. And earlier in this narrative, Karl noted how it was Schoeffel – "he was quite a philosopher," Karl said – who insisted they should regard the farmer's visit as an omen and take the problem he presented seriously.

Karl never forgot it. According to a Wausau *Daily Herald* story in February 1966 – Schoeffel was then living in Mosinee – Karl sent the $1,000 in appreciation for Schoeffel's "active participation in the development of dicumarol and warfarin."

The paper continued: "The $1,000 gift will be used by Dr. Schoeffel for the foundation of an institute for the study of the human mind."

Schoeffel expanded on his hopes for that project in an April 21, 1966, letter to Karl from Mosinee in which he thanked Karl for his "magnificent personal gift," adding, "the study of the human mind is, in essence, my future work…"

When Schoeffel died, in 1978, his news obituary in the Wausau paper noted: "Engaged in the study of the human mind, Dr. Schoeffel is credited with a bioelectronic contribution for helping amputees to work prosthetic appliances."

On June 11, 1966, Dr. Shepard Shapiro died in New York City following a long illness. As noted in this narrative, he was Elizabeth Link's brother-in-law, married to her sister, Evelyn, and a valued colleague of Karl's working on anticoagulants, in particular the use of vitamin K to counteract the anti-clotting action of dicumarol. Shapiro was buried at Forest Hill cemetery in Madison, and Karl gave a gracious tribute during the graveside rites.

In fall 1966, UW biochemistry Professor Henry Lardy – who had known and admired Karl for a quarter-century – submitted a nomination recommending Karl for the National Academy of Science's Jessie Stevenson Kovalenko Medal, awarded every two years for outstanding research in the medical sciences. The Kovalenko Fund was gifted to the National Academy in 1949 by Michael Kovalenko in memory of his wife.

Shortly after Lardy submitted Karl's nomination in November 1966, Lardy received a letter from WARF managing director Ward Ross. It showed that despite their occasional differences, Karl's relationship with UW's technology transfer unit remained strong.

Two years earlier, Karl and Ross had sparred over Karl's purported "garbage can" invention that would lure rats to traps.

But on Nov. 29, 1966, Ross wrote a letter to Lardy indicating that bruised feelings aside, WARF greatly appreciated Karl's significant contribution to both science and the foundation endowment.

"We realize... you have already submitted a nomination of Professor Link for the Kovalenko Medal," Ross wrote. "However, since our last discussion with you, we have received some very interesting information and thought we would pass it along to you regardless of whether or not you have an opportunity to use it in connection with this nomination...

"We asked our licensee, Endo Laboratories, which apparently does in excess of 80 percent of the oral anticoagulant business in the United States with its sodium warfarin product, Coumadin,

13. Doing Good for Mankind

to estimate the total number of patients treated with Coumadin since the product was introduced in 1954. Endo has come up with an estimate of 10 million patients treated with Coumadin since 1954.... We estimate that, including dicumarol, a total of 13-14 million patients in the United States have been treated with Link-discovered anticoagulants since the first one, dicumarol, was introduced on the market in 1944."

Lardy's nomination letter to Professor Harland Wood at Western Reserve University in Cleveland, chairman of the Kovalenko Fund trust committee, did not mention the Endo Lab figures, but it did a good job of listing Karl's accomplishments and earlier awards. Lardy then ended his nomination letter (which resulted in Karl being awarded the medal) with a personal note:

"As a graduate student at the University of Wisconsin, I had the privilege of learning carbohydrate chemistry from Professor Link's classroom lectures. They were brilliant; he inspired his

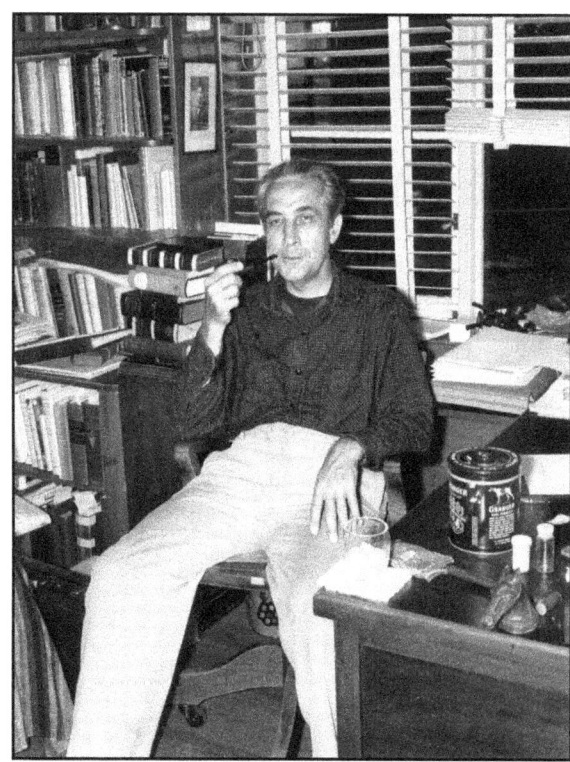

Karl at his desk in the Link family's Willow Lane home. (Link family)

students, entertained them, and encouraged even the laggards to greater achievement. We envied the students who worked directly with him, for his laboratory was by far the best equipped, it was maintained meticulously clean, and it operated around the clock. Those who achieved their Ph.D. degrees with him have gone on to brilliant individual achievements of their own. Thus, in addition to conducting outstanding research which has benefited mankind, he has been an equally outstanding teacher and has shaped the character and careers of many young men."

Karl did not go to the ceremony in Ann Arbor to receive the medal in person; Biochemistry Department chairman Robert Burris went in his place. (Conflicting reasons surfaced for Karl's absence: one suggested illness, the other an early UW seminar the very next morning that would have required a late bus from O'Hare Airport for Karl to arrive in time. In any case, the medal – solid gold and engraved "Karl Paul Link for achievement in Medical Science" – was presented to him at a Biochemistry Department gathering in Madison.)

Karl got notes of congratulations from valued colleagues, including Stanford Moore, writing from New York City, and Paul Karrer, who wrote several paragraphs – in German – from Switzerland.

For the 1967 Christmas holidays, Karl and Elizabeth welcomed sons John and Tom home to the house on Willow Lane. John and his wife Ruth brought what was now their three children (having just welcomed a son, David); Tom brought his wife, Nelly – they'd married in August – and her two children; Elizabeth's sister, Evelyn, visited as well.

In the new year, Karl continued his lifelong support of those who questioned authority and otherwise went against the grain of convention. It provided yet more evidence to counter the assertion by his colleague Robert Burris (the same Burris who traveled to Michigan for the Kovalenko medal), in his posthumous National Academy biograph of Karl, that Karl wasn't truly committed to such causes.

13. Doing Good for Mankind

On Jan. 12, 1968, Karl gave $400 to the University of Wisconsin Board of Regents "to aid students," *The Capital Times* reported, "who face difficulties because of their support of unpopular causes."

The Regents voted 6-1 to accept the gift, which was supported by UW President Fred Harrington, who said, "Prof. Link has long been interested in the defense of people who are protesting and demonstrating." The story continued: "Harrington added that Link, inventor of the rat control chemical Warfarin, has given the UW over a million dollars through gifts and royalties."

In January 1968, the *Milwaukee Journal*, Wisconsin's biggest and best newspaper, published a lengthy profile of Karl written by the talented feature writer Jay Scriba, like Karl an Indiana native.

Much of what Scriba wrote was familiar to anyone who had followed Karl's career, but a few new notes were sounded.

"I'm a bridge-builder," Karl told Scriba. "I look for relationships between scientific disciplines, as well as within biochemistry."

Karl said, "Ninety-five percent of my ideas aren't worth a damn," but added they came to him often, anytime, anywhere, and sometimes were worth recalling. "That's why I always carry a notepad and pencil."

Scriba wrote:

"Link's day usually begins about 4 a.m., when he spends an hour writing personal letters which routinely note the time, outdoor temperature and barometric pressure for the benefit of distant friends. Then, perhaps after a walk, he stuffs a couple of bananas into his briefcase and leaves his suburban home for the biochemistry building."

Scriba asked about a rumor he had heard. Did Karl really teach classes in his pajamas?

"Oh, that," Karl replied. "One morning the thermostat at home wasn't working, and I threw some things on over my pajamas and I guess I forgot to take 'em off."

Scriba added:

"It is a fact, though, that he generally strides around campus in a lumberman's wool jacket, high work shoes and a short hunting coat. He attended a medical awards luncheon in New York dressed in a red and green plaid shirt, and has been known to embellish a tuxedo with a bright red vest and buttons. (An associate declared, 'I don't think he owns a white shirt.') He is also a dynamic lecturer who once awakened a room of yawning drug manufacturers by marching to the platform with a cage containing a live chicken."

In May 1969, Karl and Elizabeth's son John climbed Mount McKinley in Alaska, the highest peak in North America, with a group of six friends.

He wrote his parents: "Our group slept in the hanger of Don Sheldon, famous mountain pilot, who is to fly us to the spot where we begin our climb."

The climbers, however, did not reach the summit after enduring a three-day storm in a snow cave at around 12,000 feet.

That fall, Karl was involved in a controversy concerning the UW Board of Regents' plan to require photo identification cards for all students, faculty, and staff. The stated reason, as reported by the *Wisconsin State Journal*, "was to cut down on the number of outside troublemakers on campus and make identification of disrupters easier."

Karl declined to participate in his scheduled Sept. 17 photo shoot, which he felt was an affront to constitutional freedoms, a decision he elaborated on in a letter to UW President Fred Harrington and Madison campus Chancellor Edwin Young.

Karl wrote that he would be "too busy" to appear for "that made-work cannery (the UW photographic unit) on Wednesday the 17th of the ninth month 1969 A.D."

He added, "I also note that staff members not on the campus during the week of Sept. 15-19 have another chance to be photographed for (a) The FBI (Mr. Hoover), (b) The Dane County sheriff, (c) The chief of the Madison police and the

13. Doing Good for Mankind

division known as Protection and Security... My reply is – non possumus (it is not possible): square it.

> "I grieve for you gentlemen.
> "I grieve for this University.
> "I grieve for this state."

The articles that appeared in *The Capital Times* and the *Wisconsin State Journal* regarding Karl's stance had an almost jocular tone; here again was the campus iconoclast, tilting at windmills. But it was more serious than that for Karl, as he wrote to an out- of-state friend, retired Denver industrial chemist W. R. Fetzer, who responded equally seriously, taking Karl to task for sympathizing with the anti-war protesters:

"The Board of Regents," Fetzer wrote, "empowered by law to govern the university, believe that a card of identity, to be carried by both faculty and students, offers some hope in that the non-student can be spotted and the student offender identified... I am of the opinion that you will lose this one BECAUSE THE OVERWHELMING PUBLIC OPINION BACKS THE REGENTS. I do not like to see your notable scientific career blackened at the end by what in my opinion is a silly evaluation of what constitutes your constitutional rights."

Karl clearly disagreed. He addressed the matter most thoughtfully in a mid-October interview with the campus newspaper *The Daily Cardinal*.

The reporter asked Karl why he was fighting the photo requirement.

"Someone has to lead the pack," Karl said. "I'm doing it by choice. I enjoy it. I love a scrap. I'm not fighting for myself. What have I got to gain? I'm concerned about the University's reputation – the one it had, has, and presumably is trying to keep. What have I got to lose – I'm damn near 70."

The *Cardinal* reporter noted that Karl paused, then added: "I could lose something more subtle. My confidence in this University. My challenge to the Regent regulation on the photo ID cards should and I hope will lead to a judicial review... That's what our courts are for. The proposition is: What are the powers of the University Regents? What are my rights as a citizen?...

"For over 40 years," Karl continued, "I have tried to work here as a scientist. But I hasten to add that in those 40 years here I have always been interested in the rights of students and the faculty. Now I am concerned about my rights as a member of the University faculty.

"In conclusion I should state that I am not in cahoots with anybody or any organization. I'm a loner. I have always been that way. But the welfare of the University faculty does concern me."

In fact, Karl was not alone in his protest of the identification cards. United Faculty – the academic union on campus – took out an advertisement saying, "We have called upon the Regents to rescind their decision, and we urge all faculty who oppose it to refuse to be photographed."

The *State Journal* reported that by early November, "nearly 2,000 faculty members on the Madison campus" had "not had their pictures taken."

The Vietnam War and the protests against it were top of mind for many as the 1960s came to an end. Karl and Elizabeth's anti-war stance was embraced by their sons, including their youngest, Paul, who as a Middleton High School student, age 16, became a decorated competitive orator early in 1970.

On March 2, Karl wrote his father-in-law, Jacob Feldman, and Jacob's wife, Rose, a letter at their winter home in Florida with the news:

"Yesterday Paul won [twice underlined] the area American Legion Oratorical contest at Cross Plains!! The next step is the state contest near Milwaukee. Paul has a really first-class speech. He might go all the way!!! It will take a first-class speech to beat him."

Karl noted that he and Elizabeth would miss the state contest, for they were headed to the West Coast to visit son Tom and his wife Nelly. Elizabeth would fly; Karl was taking the train. "I leave flying to the birds," he wrote.

13. Doing Good for Mankind

Two weeks later, young Paul Link won the statewide Legion contest, held at Central High School in West Allis. *The Capital Times* wrote that "his speech wasn't the traditional American Legion line."

Indeed it was not. Paul's speech was titled "The Erosion of Congressional War Power: A Threat to Our Democracy," and, as the *Cap Times* reported, it opposed "the practice of some American presidents of bypassing Congress in committing troops to foreign engagements."

"Link," the story noted, "hit particularly hard at the Vietnam conflict and the American involvement there."

Paul was awarded a $300 scholarship for his first-place finish, and went on to earn a Ph.D. in geology from the University of California, Santa Barbara. Paul spent four decades as a regional geologist and professor at Idaho State University.

In spring 1971, one year on from young Paul Link's winning his scholarship, the newspaper stories – front page in Madison – were about Karl. The lion of the laboratory had decided it was time to end his research career.

14. ENDGAME

THE ANNOUNCEMENT CAME May 17, the retirement effective June 30. The lead sentence from the University of Wisconsin News Service called Karl one of the school's "most distinguished, most colorful professors."

The story hit the familiar, yet enduringly impressive marks: the appearance of the farmer with the cow's blood, the long hours – years – of research, and the breakthroughs, first with anticoagulants, then the rodenticide. It spoke of his colorful dress and his willingness to speak his mind: "He has never hesitated to stand up for his beliefs, even if they caused trouble for him."

And this: "Dr. Link shared his work with his graduate students. Many of them have gone on to become famous biochemists in their own right. He is a dynamic teacher, lecturing during his career to all biochemistry majors and often coming up with surprises to illustrate his points."

One of Karl's best students, later a valued colleague and friend, Stanford Moore, won the biggest award of all, the Nobel Prize, in 1972. Moore shared the chemistry prize with Christian B. Anfinsen and William H. Stein for their research on the molecular structures of proteins.

That fall, Karl and Elizabeth traveled to Arizona to visit Karl's sister, Margaret, on her birthday.

In a short item about the visit, the *Arizona Daily Star* noted of Karl: "One of his brilliant former students, Dr. Stanford Moore, in accepting a Nobel prize this summer for his pioneering research in enzymes, said in his acceptance, 'If there is one man

14. ENDGAME

to thank it is Karl P. Link… he is the man who formed most of my career.'"

In retirement, Karl continued to make news – or at least he was still sought out by reporters looking for a story. The *Daily Cardinal*'s Summer Registration issue in 1973 included an interview with Karl under the headline: "Link: the scientist as radical."

The story began, "Karl Paul Link is a rare academic achievement: a successful combination of non-conformist leftism and outstanding scientific accomplishments."

The Watergate scandal had just begun to be exposed, and Karl weighed in with his opinion of President Richard Nixon (who had been treated with warfarin for his phlebitis), variously describing Nixon as a "vindictive son of a bitch," a "bastard" and "slippery as an eel."

"To think that guy had the guts to campaign on law and order," Karl told the *Cardinal*. "What a crook."

Locally, however, Karl felt the election of a young, progressive mayor in spring 1973 was a highly positive sign: "The best thing that ever happened to Madison is the election of [Paul] Soglin."

The *Cardinal* reporter ended the story by quoting Karl on his team that had revolutionized anticoagulants: "I think the secret of their success is three-pronged," he said. "They never ceased to wonder, they kept on trying, and they were on a project directed toward doing mankind some good instead of trying to destroy it."

Not unexpectedly, Karl's favorite Madison newspaper reporter, the *State Journal*'s John Newhouse, caught up with him for a retirement piece in March 1974.

Just prior, Karl and Elizabeth had taken a trip to England, for a dinner to honor Dr. A. C. Chibnall, a member of the Royal Society of London, the United Kingdom's national academy of sciences.

The event was held at Cambridge University and included dinner in a formal dining hall with the unlikely name of the Old

Kitchen. Chibnall, Karl told Newhouse upon their return, had "produced four Nobel prize winners. I've only produced one."

At the Cambridge dinner, Karl found himself seated next to Sir Rudolph Peters, a decorated British biochemist and one of the world's leading experts on vitamin B and carbohydrate metabolism.

Link told Newhouse that he and Peters enjoyed a spirited conversation in which Karl talked about two compounds he'd recently been experimenting with. Being Karl, he referred to them as his Secret Elixir and his Super-Secret Elixir.

(In a later letter to UW-Madison archivist Bernie Schermetzler, Newhouse wrote this about Karl's Secret Elixir: "It was dried yeast and Vitamin C – nothing more. He prescribed it for my wife's arthritis and it seemed to help. The Super-Secret Elixir was something else.")

In England, Karl revealed to Peters some details of his Super-Secret Elixir, which he said could ease pain and promote longevity.

Karl shared Peters' reply with Newhouse: "Link, the ordinary biochemist would think you're a quack, but – do you know – I think you're a notch ahead on something we've missed over here."

In his letter to the UW-Madison archivist after Karl's death, Newhouse mused about Karl's Super-Secret Elixir. Did it exist? Newhouse thought it might.

"He told me," Newhouse wrote, "that as a boy back in Indiana, there was a little Irish ditch digger who suffered horribly with arthritis and who got into some yeasty waste fluid from the local brewery and was transformed into a terrific ditch digger. Sang and dug ditches like crazy.

"And then there was a delivery wagon horse, arthritic – apparently – as could be. He leaned over the brewery fence, lapped up some of the yeasty stuff, and became a young horse again. Hence Karl figured there was something valuable in the brewery waste yeast – much like the dicumarol and Warfarin he extracted from spoiled sweet clover hay.

14. Endgame

"Karl became a consultant for the Pabst Brewing Company, and... worked on a new yeast with great promise."

In his letter, Newhouse notes that Karl's contact at Pabst eventually died and that the brewery attorneys were not impressed with his work on the Super-Secret Elixir. Newhouse asked Karl where things stood.

"He did the usual kidding and stalling," Newhouse wrote. But he added, "I am haunted by the idea that he may really have had something. He referred to adding something to the diet of the yeast to make it the superior product."

Newhouse ended his March 1974 piece on Karl with this: "Link figures he has time to continue work on the Super-Secret Elixir. He comes from a hardy line."

He closed with a quote from Karl: "Brother Ted – he's 77 and I'm 73 – watched Halley's Comet from the roof of our house in 1910. It's coming back in 1985. I plan on seeing it again."

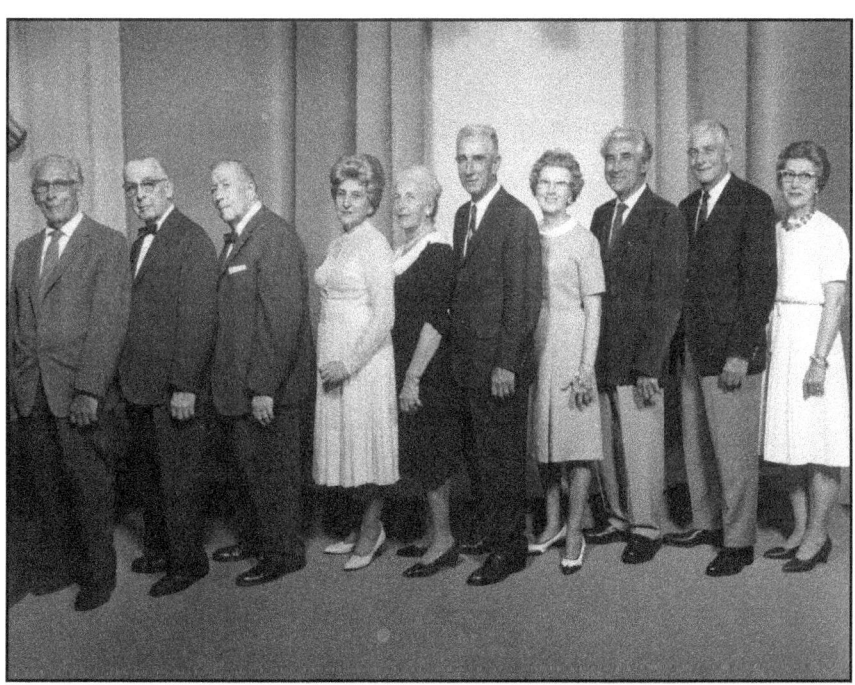

The Link siblings, left to right, in a later photo: George, Alfred, Herbert, Helene, Ruth, Theodore, Agnes, Karl, Walter, and Margaret. (Link family)

"Brother George – here's his picture, in the *National Geographic* magazine – is a tough nut. He's 86. He goes mountaineering every year, falls off some rocks, stays in bed a week, and starts out again.

"Sister Helene is 81. We write every week. She tells people that I did a wonderful thing, made it possible for rats to die without feeling any pain."

Karl's self-prognosis, alas, proved inaccurate. He suffered two heart attacks early in 1975, each requiring an extended hospital stay. Yet he bounced back. By late March, he was home on Willow Lane, where a public health nurse from the Visiting Nurse Service visited twice a week to take his blood pressure, check vital signs and help Elizabeth with his medication schedule.

A *Capital Times* reporter doing a story on the nurse service visited and reported Karl "looks healthy and his spirits are high, surrounded by friends and family and a faithful dog. Link's eyes sparkle when he says, 'I plan to live until Halley's Comet returns… and then some.'"

On October 23, 1975, Elizabeth's father, Jacob Feldman, died in a hospital in Miami Beach. A news story about his death that appeared in *The Capital Times* noted he'd been a prominent Madison businessman, owner of the Feldman Grocery Store and Feldman Paper Box Co., as well as a member of the Madison Rotary Club for nearly 50 years. Karl ironically noted that Jacob was "The Bolshevik Rotarian," reminiscent of his political activism in Poland and his business success in Madison.

Karl was still reading newspapers, clipping items that interested him, and writing letters to the editor. During his morning walks, he would occasionally annotate the morning newspaper of a neighbor family in the Highlands who advocated for environmental conservation.

In August 1976, he wrote a note to *Capital Times* editor Miles McMillin, with a reference to an anniversary a year earlier of a bombing in Japan. It speaks one last time to Karl's decades-long activism against not only atomic and nuclear weapons but all manner of nuclear power.

14. Endgame

McMillin wrote: "Karl Paul Link favors me with this excellent quote from the 'Scientific Declaration on Nuclear Power,' presented to the Congress and the President of the United States on the 30th anniversary of the bombing of Hiroshima and signed by more than 2,000 biologists, chemists, engineers and other scientists:

"'The country must recognize that it now appears imprudent to move forward with a rapidly expanding nuclear power plant construction program. The risks of doing so are altogether too great. We, therefore, urge a drastic reduction in new nuclear power plant construction starts before major progress is achieved in the required research and in resolving present controversies about safety, waste disposal, and plutonium safeguards. For similar reasons, we urge the nation to suspend its program of exporting nuclear plants to other countries pending resolution of the national security questions associated with the use by these countries of the by-product plutonium from United States reactors.'"

Two months after sending the quote to McMillin, Karl experienced difficulty breathing in the early hours of Sunday, Oct. 24, 1976. An ambulance was dispatched to Willow Lane and Karl was taken to Madison General Hospital, where his condition was listed as "satisfactory." By Wednesday, a *State Journal* headline read: "Biochemist Karl Link 'improved.'" He left the hospital within a few days, but his hopes for an encore viewing of Halley's Comet, still a decade away, were clearly not bright.

Karl was well enough in March 1978 to make a trip to Tucson for a family gathering. Present were his older brother George and their sisters Helene, Ruth, Agnes, and Margaret. Karl's son Tom and his son, Paco, were there as well, from their home in Eugene, Oregon.

"I wished I had a tape recorder," Tom Link said, recalling seeing his father in Tucson. "He was clear as a bell and remembered everything, and that wasn't always the case [toward the end]."

Everyone attended services at Tucson's Grace Episcopal Church, where Helene, now 85 and a former director of the church choir, stepped in as guest director and – according to sister Margaret – "nearly brought the walls down."

The family had assembled to celebrate George's 90th birthday, a milestone he reached March 14. George had lived in Tucson since 1956 and – in the accomplished manner of the Link siblings – enjoyed a distinguished career as a botanist. George's hobbies also spoke of accomplishment. He mapped trails and blazed new ones in Yoho National Park in the Canadian Rockies – 32 in all. He also spent decades translating the works of the Greek botanist Theophrastus.

In May 1978, Karl received an honorary membership to the Wisconsin Academy of Arts and Sciences, inducted along with author and environmentalist Sigurd Olson and Nobel Prize winning oncology researcher and UW professor Howard Temin.

Karl's sister, Ruth Link, died June 4 in Tucson, age 83. She was the third of Karl's siblings to die in the past decade. Brothers Alfred and Herbert both died in La Porte, Alfred, a noted lawyer, in 1972, and Herbert, who served as an official U.S. Weather Bureau observer, in 1969.

On Nov. 22, 1978, Karl Paul Link died, at home in the Highlands neighborhood where he and Elizabeth had lived for decades.

"As far as I know," his son, Tom Link, said, "he suffered a stroke and died immediately."

Karl's death was page one news in both Madison's *Capital Times* and *Wisconsin State Journal*. The stories detailed his scientific discoveries and the honors they brought and recalled his flamboyance and irreverence.

UW System President Edwin Young issued a statement: "We have lost one of the most brilliant scientists we have ever had at the University of Wisconsin. He was a great man and a man who loved to deflate the egos of administrators, myself included. I am very saddened."

14. Endgame

Hector DeLuca, who took a graduate course from Link and in 1978 was chairman of the Biochemistry Department, said, "He was a superb teacher, one of the best lecturers this department or this university ever had."

The *Capital Times* abetted its news obituary with an editorial: "His death has taken from the campus and this community a brilliant scholar and researcher."

Friends and colleagues, too, reacted with sadness mixed with warm and sometimes humorous memories.

Karl's Nobel Prize-winning former student, Stanford Moore, sent a Western Union telegram from New York City to Elizabeth Link: "Karl was a great teacher and friend whose contribution to my career will always be cherished. The opportunity to talk to him a month ago gave me an occasion to let him know again how much I appreciated his friendship. My expression of my feeling of loss is addressed to all of the members of the Link family."

Another of Karl's students, Clint Ballou, wrote Elizabeth a note of condolence:

"The telephone call from Collin Schroeder [also a student of Karl's] about Karl shook me even though I had been expecting it to come. Then I recalled all the good times we had together at Madison, and most of the sadness went away.

"When I arrived in Madison as a beginning student," Ballou continued, "it was perplexing to find that Karl was not available to advise me (he was in the sanitorium across the lake). However, it soon became apparent that he exerted an influence even from such a distance, and throughout my graduate years his direction was there even though it was not always obvious. I think I learned a lot about how to deal with my own students from that experience. He molded a person even while giving the freedom to grow as an individual. It took a delicate touch, but it was the most important time of my life."

Ballou subsequently contributed an article about Karl's scientific achievement to the journal *Advances in Carbohydrate Chemistry and Biochemistry*. The piece is detailed in its scientific jargon, but also captures Karl's genius for teaching and his colorful personality. It is worth quoting at length:

"Perhaps the clearest influence that Link exerted was in his teaching of carbohydrate chemistry, or, in modern terminology...'carbohydrate chemistry and society.' His formal teaching was factual and descriptive, as might be expected, but it was never dull or uninteresting. With the chalk board of full of detailed reactions describing the interconversions of the hexoses, written in a precise and careful hand well before the class began, he then had time to sketch the 'personality' of science as he related the important facts concerning the follies of mankind.

"Of the 55 doctoral candidates whom Link supervised, over 30 worked partly or wholly on carbohydrates. Life in the laboratory was centered around the regular, Friday lab cleanup and research conference. To perform poorly in either activity was something to be avoided. In research conferences, Link aimed to help rather than embarrass...

"Link was impressive in both appearance and demeanor. He projected a size that exceeded his real physical dimensions. His casual dress conveyed the air of a relaxed country squire completely at ease in a formal and distrustful world. A well-worn black herringbone-tweed jacket, flannel shirt, large knotted tie, and unpressed grey trousers were usually accompanied by a wide-brimmed hat, and brown work-shoes suited for tramping the countryside as well as the halls of academia. His somewhat swarthy features and long flowing hair added to the image, intended or not, of a character actor, and he once confided that he might have had a successful career on the stage had he chosen acting instead of science. In any event, one sensed that he was always 'on stage' and was aware of an obligation to pique or stimulate the audience...

"It is not a happy moment," Ballou concluded, "when writing on the passing of a close friend, colleague, and mentor. In this instance, the sadness is tempered by the recognition that Karl Link had a long, creative, productive, and eminently successful

14. Endgame

life. He left his mark on science, and he left it on the people who knew him and on the many who had only heard his name. The farmers of Wisconsin probably recognized his true worth better than any others, and it was their judgment he valued most. But the medical profession was generous in its praise, and his students and the general public will not forget."

Clint Ballou's wife, Dorothy Lun Wu, also a former student of Karl's, wrote a separate note of condolence to Elizabeth:

"I thought we were prepared to understand that life is but a walk on earth. We came, and we will have to leave. But when this happens to someone close to us, someone we dearly love, someone who has loved us, taught us, given us wisdom and vision and courage, we are at a loss."

Robert Bock, Dean of the UW-Madison Graduate School, wrote Elizabeth: "Please accept my deepest sympathy. I am one of many persons whose life has been made more worthwhile because of Karl Paul Link.

"I was a student in his seminar course, attended many of his stimulating lectures and felt welcome in the Department because of his sincere interest in students.

"I became a faculty member and his colleague, enjoyed the excitement of joint research projects on calf scours, dicumarol and carbohydrate structure. When I became an administrator, his humor via post cards or a chat in the corridor served to remind me of my responsibility and mission. I deeply appreciate the flattery of this great scientist cheering me on or advising me to try a fresh tack. He added much to many lives including mine. I will miss my dear friend and colleague."

And from the memorial resolution from Karl's UW-Madison faculty colleagues:

"Students on the Madison campus found in Karl Paul Link a stimulating teacher, a friend, and an advocate. Unconventional in dress and outspoken on current issues, he lectured with a theatrical flair that could be matched by few of his colleagues. Outside the classroom he was a staunch defender of the students' right to freedom of expression, whether or not he approved of the causes they were supporting. His commitment to civil liberties is illustrated by his willingness to serve as faculty advisor to a left-wing student organization during the dark days of McCarthyism, and many other instances of his active opposition to a sometimes oppressive establishment could be cited.

"Karl Paul Link is remembered with affection by over 70 graduate students who worked for the M.S. or Ph.D. degree under his direction. He frequently emphasized the group nature of scientific research and achievement, but he had a keen appreciation of each student's unique potential, and a gift for fostering the realization of that potential. While demanding nothing less than their best performance he taught his students the joy of scientific discovery, and thus sustained them in learning their difficult craft. Now he is gone, but he has left behind the indelible mark of his own uniqueness."

A memorial service for Karl was held May 27, 1979, at the First Unitarian Meeting House in Madison.

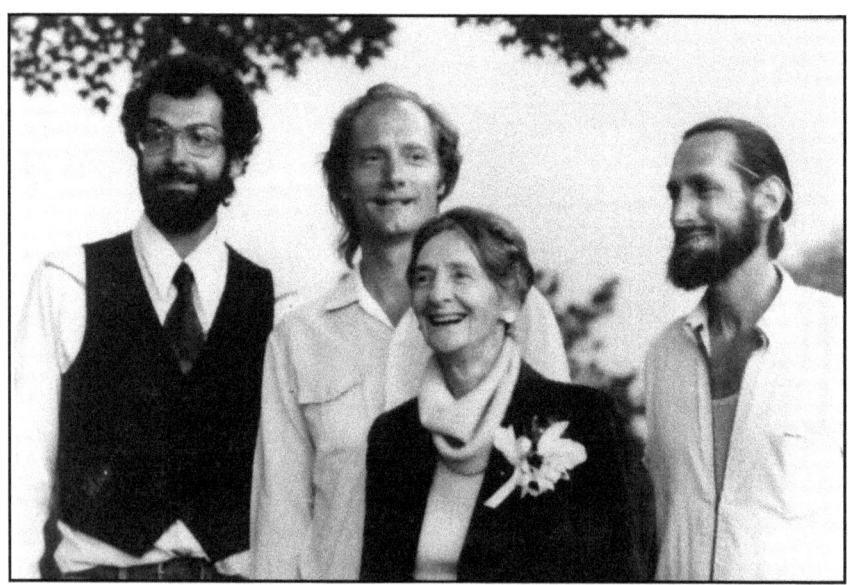

Paul, Tom, Elizabeth and John Link at Karl's memorial service. (Link family)

14. Endgame

In his biographical essay on Karl, Robert Burris noted, "The memorial was a joyful occasion as Karl would have wanted. There were tributes by his family, his students, faculty members, and other friends."

Twenty months after Karl died, John Kailin Link, Karl and Elizabeth's first son, died in an August 1980 mountain accident in Colorado. The fall occurred at the base of The Cleaver in the Wild Basin area of Rocky Mountain National Park. John was training for the Pikes Peak Marathon, a race he had competed in four times and won first place twice in his age class. A dedicated long-distance trail runner, including up and down volcanos in Mexico, and triathlete, John had lived in Boulder since 1966 and died at age 43. He was survived by his four children, Lisa, Andrea, David, and Mara.

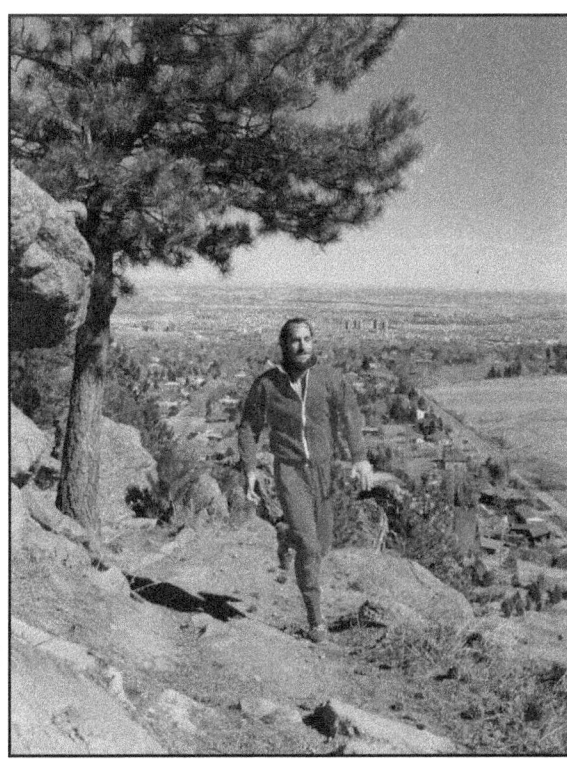

John Link trail running in Boulder, Colorado, circa late 1970s. (Link family)

Elizabeth Link, meanwhile, was fighting bone cancer, and succumbed April 24, 1982, age 74.

The *Capital Times* took note in an editorial:

"Elizabeth (Lisa) Link may not have been as well known as her late husband, Karl Paul Link, the brilliant University of Wisconsin biochemist. But Mrs. Link, who died last week at the age of 74, left and enduring legacy of love and social commitment.

"Mrs. Link was at the forefront of the movement for peace and disarmament long before it had achieved the broad base of support it enjoys today. A tireless marcher and petition signer, she helped found the local chapter of the Women's International League for Peace and Freedom and actively promoted friendship between the U.S. and Soviet people.

"Even in her last days, while confined to her bed, she was circulating petitions in favor of a nuclear weapons freeze."

On April 1, 1982, a little more than three weeks before she died, Elizabeth dictated a message stating her desire for the Willow Lane home she shared with Karl to be used as a meeting place for those promoting peace.

"I wish this home to remain forever as a peace house," Elizabeth said.

Elizabeth originally hoped the Jane Addams Peace Association would take residence in the home, but according to a news account the group "decided that the home is too small for their needs."

Instead, the home went to the Society of Friends, known as Quakers, and they brought in Sister Betty Richardson, a Catholic nun, to promote what was being called "Link House" as a training center and retreat for peace groups. In addition, in 1983, the city of Madison created the Elizabeth (Lisa) Link Peace Park adjacent to State Street downtown.

14. Endgame

The plaques in the park include the following tributes to Elizabeth:

> "Founded in 1915, the Women's International League for Peace and Freedom works toward world disarmament and establishing political, social and economic conditions that assure freedom, justice and peace for all. Lisa Link was at the heart of WILPF for 30 years until her death in 1982."

A quote from Elizabeth is also prominently displayed:

> "My wish for each of you is that the peace and freedom we have all worked so earnestly to achieve will indeed find reality with human beings loving and cherishing each another the world over."

Just a few weeks after Elizabeth died, an extraordinary gathering was held in a clearing on the wooded lot of the Link home in the Highlands. People came – and they numbered nearly 200 – to honor Elizabeth and her lifelong, tireless commitment to peace and social justice.

Don Behm, a Milwaukee journalist who earlier wrote an extended biographical essay on Karl, did a story on Elizabeth for the Madison weekly newspaper, *Isthmus*, which ran it on the cover with the headline: "A Peacemaker's Legacy."

Behm interviewed numerous friends and colleagues of Elizabeth, including her Highlands neighbor, Barbara Davis, who recalled that earlier in the year Elizabeth had returned from a trip to New York for medical treatment, and on landing in Madison, was taken by ambulance to a Madison hospital for further care.

"By the time she had arrived at the hospital," Davis said, "she had convinced the driver and the attendant to sign her nuclear disarmament petition."

The local chapter of the Women's International League for Peace and Freedom – which Elizabeth helped found – gave her its

"Peace and Freedom Award" for the second time at their annual dinner in late April, the month Elizabeth died.

She'd composed a note of appreciation and encouragement that was read at the dinner:

"My ability to accept [this honor] comes from knowing that only through our persistent effort can we together achieve the ends we all hold so dear. I become merely a symbol for all of you, and we shall overcome…It is only with all of you that I could do whatever I have been able to do for peace."

An Elizabeth and Karl Paul Link Lecture was established on the UW-Madison campus, and in April 1985, it was delivered in the auditorium of the Wisconsin Historical Society by Victor Weisskopf, an emeritus professor at MIT and founder of the Federation of Atomic Scientists, an organization dedicated to outlining the potential peril of nuclear arms.

In the late 1980s, Link House became the Link Friendship House, under the direction of Ed Durkin, a retired Madison fire chief. Durkin led delegations on trips to China and the Soviet Union, and Russia after the USSR's dissolution.

He also hosted delegations from those countries at the Link Friendship House. The most memorable may have occurred in 1992. A group of Soviet cosmonauts was coming to the United States and as part of the trip would be attending the celebrated air show held annually in Oshkosh, some 80 miles from Madison.

Durkin located the trip organizers and offered some money toward expenses. In return, the cosmonauts would spend a couple of days in Madison, which they did, in August 1992. Durkin found private residences for three of the cosmonauts while the fourth, Sergei Krikalev, and his wife, Elena Terekhina, stayed with Durkin at the Link Friendship House.

Krikalev, who spoke good English, addressed the Madison Downtown Rotary. His remarks drew press coverage, and a subsequent invitation to visit NASA.

Less than two years later, Krikalev became the first Russian ever invited aboard a U.S. Space Shuttle. He was able to invite a

14. ENDGAME

few people to witness the launch at Kennedy Space Center, and Durkin was one.

"Even though you are three miles away," Durkin said later, "there is no way TV does it justice. The noise is deafening. You can feel the heat. The earth rumbles. All my volunteering, all my work over 15 years, was made totally worthwhile in those three minutes."

In the early 1990s, a University of Wisconsin mathematics professor named Anatole Beck initiated an effort to get Campus Drive, a street on the west end of the UW-Madison campus, renamed Karl Paul Link Drive. It was an inspired choice of streets, in that Campus Drive runs past buildings that were important in Karl's career, including WARF tower, the Biochemistry building, the Stock Pavilion and UW Hospital and Clinics.

Beck had witnessed an earlier 1980s effort – spearheaded by a Madison morning radio host – to get Campus Drive renamed for the former UW athletic director Elroy "Crazylegs" Hirsch. Various bureaucracies signed off, but when the cost for new signs was publicized – somewhere north of $17,000 – the idea was scaled back and a small section of Oakland Avenue, near the football stadium, was renamed Crazylegs Lane.

Beck recalled the Crazylegs saga when, in 1992, Hirsch had a major heart operation and was prescribed warfarin. Beck reasoned the man who was the driving force behind the revolutionary human anticoagulant and rodenticide was as deserving – or more so – of a street name recognition as a sports star.

"We had a great man living among us whose memory has virtually been erased," Beck told Isthmus.

Beck felt he could get university or WARF funding – the cost now estimated at $20,000 – for the new signs, but it was not forthcoming.

A few years later, Karl's son, Tom Link, got on board, and elicited support from Biochemistry Department chairman and decorated scientist Hector DeLuca.

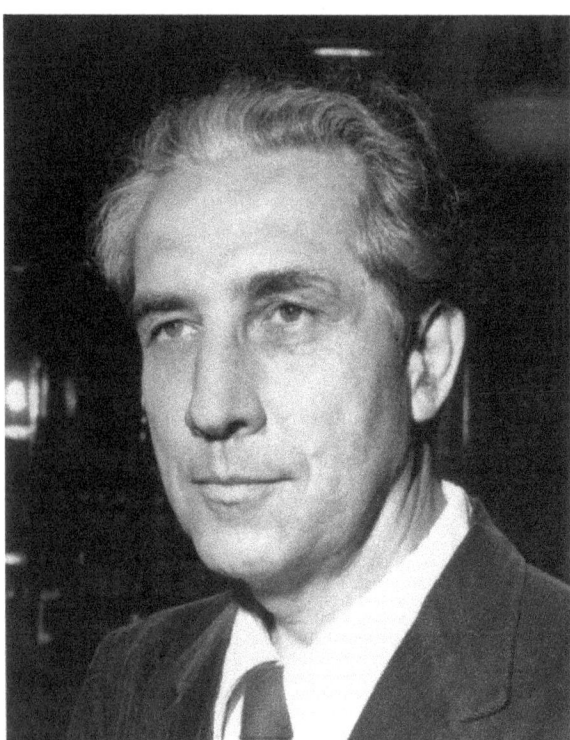

Karl Paul Link.
(UW-Madison Archive)

"I am in total support of naming Campus Drive Karl Paul Link Drive," DeLuca wrote in a July 21, 1997, letter to Tom.

That endorsement may have led WARF and UW officials to change their minds. A story in *Isthmus* reported the money was secured. But then another problem emerged, as *Isthmus* noted: "The plan is facing another roadblock: the opposition of University Avenue businesses, who fear the name will create confusion."

It was largely one business, at the west end of Campus Drive (but without a Campus Drive address), that raised a ruckus. It was enough. Karl Paul Link Drive was tabled again.

A decade on, Anatole Beck was back, proposing the street name change to the UW Faculty Senate. Referencing the continued societal benefits provided by warfarin, Beck said of Karl to the *Wisconsin State Journal* in 2008:

"This is a man who has been dead for [30] years, and he's still out there slaying dragons for us."

14. ENDGAME

Once again, Beck's efforts fell short. Campus Drive is still Campus Drive in Madison.

Yet Karl's achievement continues to resonate. On Jan. 30, 2008, UW biochemistry Professor David Nelson and Karl's son, Tom, gave a "Wednesday Night at the Lab" presentation on campus honoring the 75th anniversary of the day the Wisconsin farmer, Ed Carlson, showed up in Madison with cow's blood and spoiled sweet clover and met Karl Paul Link, a meeting that led to one of the more consequential medical discoveries of the 20th century.

It was a fascinating night. Nelson and Tom Link had attended graduate school together at Stanford University. Nelson first met Karl when Karl came to visit Tom in Palo Alto, always with an armload of *Proceedings of the National Academy of Sciences* journals in hand.

During their 2008 program together, Nelson handled the description of Karl's scientific accomplishments, while Tom shared personal anecdotes with his children Syon, Acaya, and Sundara in attendance.

Toward the end of his part of the presentation, after detailing the evolution of the anticoagulants that were central to Karl's science, Nelson noted that the flamboyance of Karl's personality – which charmed some and irritated others – might well have helped the science.

"Link was something of a showman," Nelson said, "and was able to publicize his work in a way that was good for everybody. We scientists need to do that better."

Nelson continued: "We don't tell the public what we have to offer them. Link did that, that's for sure."

Concluding, Nelson said: "We're talking about somebody here who was a tremendous scientist. Nobody has any question about that. He was one of the first people to really straddle the chasm between academic research and commercial applications of that research."

Tom Link said that if he was going to be honest – and he was – Karl did not have a lot of time for conventional parenting.

"He was preoccupied," Tom said, "with promoting warfarin and dicumarol and with his teaching and encounters with university administrators."

Which did not mean they didn't have fine times together.

"He had a wonderfully warm and compelling personality," Tom said of his father. "When we went out, I became transformed from this rather shy and average child into somebody who was very important. I was his helper."

Tom recalled "a beautiful spring day in 1957" when he came home from track practice and – at 16 – was offered a shot of bourbon by his father, who said they were celebrating. Tom asked what had happened.

"Joe McCarthy died," Karl said.

As he concluded, Tom noted how in Robert Burris's biographical essay about Karl, Burris had suggested that Karl was not truly a great defender of liberal and unpopular causes.

"I very strongly disagree," Tom said. "One of the most interesting things about Karl is that he really wanted to make a difference. He wasn't willing to limit that to science. He took political stands over the years and was criticized by some for it."

It was noted above that Karl's achievements in the lab continue to resonate. In October 2022, approaching the 90th anniversary of Karl's first encounter with the distraught Wisconsin farmer and bucket of cow blood, the American Chemical Society (ACS) recognized the invention of warfarin as a National Historic Chemical Landmark, a designation that was launched in 1992 to honor significant achievements in the history of chemistry.

At the time of the announcement, ACS President Angela K. Wilson said, "Warfarin has helped millions of patients lessen the risk of stroke or heart attack. It has also been used as a rat poison that has reduced the spread of rodent-borne diseases. In addition, proceeds from the associated patents are important contributors to

14. Endgame

other research funded by WARF at the University of Wisconsin-Madison."

An accompanying news release noted that warfarin "remains one of the most widely used treatments for blood clots to this day. Experts estimate that around 100 million prescriptions of warfarin are still issued globally each year."

A groundbreaking ceremony for warfarin's landmark status was held in a new courtyard in a greenspace between the three buildings in the Hector DeLuca Biochemical Sciences Complex on the University of Wisconsin-Madison campus. A bronze plaque recognizing the honor will be mounted on a wall of the courtyard.

What would Karl Paul Link make of such a prestigious honor? Certainly, he'd be pleased – though perhaps wondering why it took so long. Whatever the reaction, there would be a twinkle in his eye. Before long he'd be asking if they'd ever heard the story of farmer Ed Carlson.

THE END

ACKNOWLEDGMENTS

THIS BOOK'S GENESIS, many years ago, came with a visit to the Madison offices of *The Capital Times* newspaper, where I was writing a daily column, by Tom Link, Karl Paul Link's son.

He'd brought notes, letters, and scrapbooks, and wondered if I might have interest in writing a book about his father, who died in 1978.

I knew that Karl Paul Link was a celebrated scientist, and that he had a colorful personality, but I was writing five newspaper columns a week at the time and although I'd done a couple of books, I didn't immediately sign on to Tom's project.

Years later – a decade? – I'd left the newspaper business, or it had left me, and I reached back to Tom. Was he still interested in that book?

Tom was interested. From day one, or even, as noted, before day one, Tom was the driving force behind this book. He was endlessly encouraging, opening doors, and sharing family correspondence and memorabilia. This book would not exist without him.

A few other people deserved special mention and thanks. David Nelson, Professor Emeritus of Biochemistry at the University of Wisconsin-Madison, was enormously helpful, granting an extended interview and then answering follow up questions. It was Nelson who helped organize Karl's substantial archive, housed at UW Archives in Steenbock Library on the UW-Madison campus, which includes voluminous correspondence, as well as dozens of pages of Karl's unfinished memoir. Dave read and commented on an early draft of the manuscript as well. The archivists themselves were unfailingly helpful in finding the appropriate boxes for each of my research visits, as well as several images from Karl's archive which appear in the text.

Kevin Walters, a public affairs analyst at the Wisconsin Alumni Research Association (WARF) and a historian unmatched in his knowledge of WARF, also granted an interview and read and commented on the manuscript.

Andrea K. Banks, Karl's granddaughter – her father was Karl's oldest son, John – volunteered a great deal of time to reading and commenting on the manuscript, locating and sourcing photographs, and otherwise helping make the book the best it could be.

My friend Dee Grimsrud helped trace the genealogy of the Link family, genealogy being something she has done for a number of my books. But for this book, Dee's research skills were also able to confirm the presence of a young farmer in St. Croix County, Wisconsin, in 1933 – Ed Carlson, who arrived in Madison with blood from his dying cows, kicking off Karl Paul Link's research into anticoagulants.

The Link family would like to thank Joyal Holder with Holder Printworks for all his guidance, patience, and assistance in digitizing the family collection of photos and archives. Thanks as well to the Harry S. Truman Presidential Library and Museum for information regarding the 1955 Lasker Awards ceremony.

For personal interviews, thanks to Tom Link; Dave Nelson; Kevin Walters; Joan Link Coles, daughter of Karl's brother, Walter; Sandra Lignell, daughter of Karl's brother, Herbert; Hector DeLuca, esteemed UW-Madison scientist; and two of Karl's students from the 1960s: Walt Barker and Mark Hermodson.

Dr. Marcia Richards, the daughter of Karl's colleague Mark Stahmann, kindly invited me into her home and allowed me to photocopy her father's correspondence, which helped me provide Stahmann's side of the unfortunate fracturing of his relationship with Karl Paul Link.

Acknowledgements

Other sources are credited in the text itself, including University of Wisconsin Oral History Program interviews with Henry Lardy, Anne Terrio, and Harold Campbell; an American Medical Society "Men and Molecules" radio interview; biographical essays on Karl Paul Link written by Robert Burris and Don Behm; "The Discovery of Dicumarol and Its Sequels," a 1959 article in the journal *Circulation* adapted from Karl Paul Link's speech in New York City a year earlier; an unpublished history of WARF by Clay Schoenfeld; an essay in the journal *Advances in Carbohydrate Chemistry and Biochemistry* on Karl Paul Link's scientific achievements, written by Karl's former student Clint Ballou; and numerous newspaper and magazine articles, especially the Madison newspapers *The Capital Times* and *Wisconsin State Journal*, which, helpfully for the biographer, found Karl Paul Link to make excellent copy.

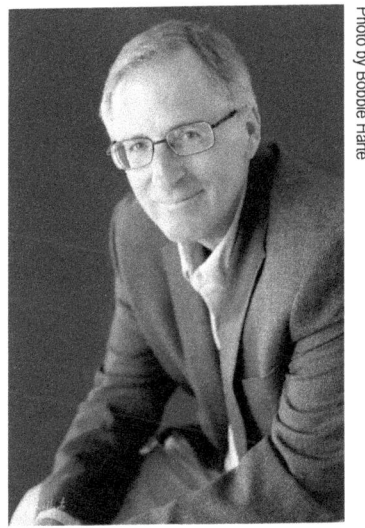

ABOUT THE AUTHOR

Doug Moe has worked as a journalist in Wisconsin for more than four decades. He has authored more than a dozen books, including most recently, "Moments of Happiness: A Wisconsin Band Story," a collaboration with Mike Leckrone on the legendary band leader's autobiography.

Please visit www.dougmoe.org for more information.

www.ingramcontent.com/pod-product-compliance
Lightning Source LLC
Chambersburg PA
CBHW050029090426
42735CB00021B/3422